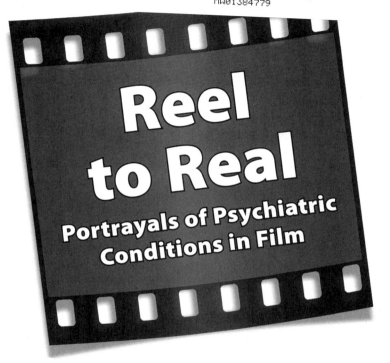

Reel to Real
Portrayals of Psychiatric Conditions in Film

David J. Robinson, MD, FRCPC
Fellow of the American Psychiatric Association

***Reel to Real:* Psychiatric Conditions in Cinema**

Rapid Psychler® Press

Suite 374
3560 Pine Grove Ave.
Port Huron, Michigan
USA 48060

Suite 203
1673 Richmond St.
London, Ontario
Canada N6G 2N3

Toll Free Phone   888-PSY-CHLE (888-779-2453)
Toll Free Fax   888-PSY-CHLR (888-779-2457)
Outside the U.S. & Canada — Fax 519-675-0610
website   www.psychler.com
email   rapid@psychler.com

ISBN (13) 978-1-894328-29-6, (10) 1-894328-29-9
© 2009, Rapid Psychler Press, First Edition
Printed in the United States of America

All rights reserved. This book is protected by copyright. No part of this book may be reproduced in any form or by any means without express written permission. Unauthorized copying is prohibited by law and will be dealt with by a punitive superego as well as all available legal means (including a lawyer with a Cluster B Personality Disorder). Please support the creative process by not photocopying this book.

All caricatures are fictitious. Any resemblance to real people, either living or deceased, is entirely coincidental (and unfortunate). The author assumes no responsibility for the consequences of diagnoses made, or treatment instituted, as a result of the contents of this book. Qualified mental health professionals should make such determinations. Every effort was made to ensure that the information in this book was accurate at the time of publication. Due to the changing nature of the field of psychiatry, the reader is encouraged to consult both additional, and more recent, sources of information.

Dedication & Acknowledgments

Dedication
This book is dedicated to my "Russian sister"

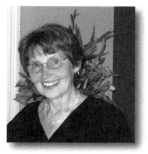

Dr. Lyudmila Burdan

Acknowledgments
- Jennifer Robinson
- Monty & Lil Robinson
- Brian & Brenda Chapman
- Sue Fletcher-Keron and Randy Keron
- Brad Groshok & Susan McFarland

Rapid Psychler® Press 🚲
produces books and presentation media that are:
- comprehensively researched
- well organized
- formatted for ease of use
- reasonably priced
- clinically oriented, and
- include humor that enhances education, and that neither demeans patients nor the efforts of those who treat them.

Reel to Real: Psychiatric Conditions in Cinema

Table of Contents

Dedication	3
Differences Between *Reel to Real* and *Reel Psychiatry*	8
Movie Rating System	10
Disclaimers	10
Format Used in *Reel to Real*	14

1. Psychotic Disorders

Schizophrenia: Disorganized Type	15
Schizophrenia: Catatonic Type	16
Schizophrenia: Paranoid Type	17
Schizophrenia: Undifferentiated Type	18
Schizophreniform Disorder	19
Schizoaffective Disorder	20
Delusional Disorder: Erotomanic Type	21
Delusional Disorder: Grandiose Type	22
Delusional Disorder: Infidelity/Jealous Type	23
Delusional Disorder: Paranoid Type	24
Delusional Disorder: Somatic Type	25
Shared Psychotic Disorder	26

2. Mood Disorders

Major Depressive Disorder: Severe With Psychotic Features	27
Major Depressive Disorder: Severe Without Psychotic Features	28
Major Depressive Disorder: Single Episode, Moderate	29
Dysthymic Disorder	30
Bipolar I Disorder: Severe With Psychotic Features	31
Bipolar I Disorder: Severe Without Psychotic Features	32
Bipolar I Disorder: Moderate	33
Cyclothymic Disorder	34

3. Anxiety Disorders

Panic Disorder	35
Agoraphobia	36
Posttraumatic Stress Disorder	37
Obsessive-Compulsive Disorder	38
Generalized Anxiety Disorder	39
Specific Phobias	40
Social Phobia	41

Table of Contents

4. Somatoform Disorders
Hypochondriasis	42
Conversion Disorder	43
Body Dysmorphic Disorder	44

5. Factitious Disorder and Malingering
Factitious Disorder	45
Malingering	46

6. Dissociative Disorders
Dissociative Identity Disorder	47
Dissociative Fugue	48

7. Sexual and Gender Identity Disorders
Pedophilia	49
Sexual Masochism and Sexual Sadism	50
Transvestic Fetishism	51
Voyeurism	52
Gender Identity Disorder	53

8. Eating Disorders
Anorexia Nervosa	54
Bulimia Nervosa	55

9. Sleep Disorders
Primary Insomnia	56
Narcolepsy	57
Circadian Rhythm Sleep Disorder	58
Nightmare Disorder	59
Sleepwalking Disorder	60

10. Impulse-Control Disorders
Intermittent Explosive Disorder	61
Kleptomania	62
Pathological Gambling	63
Pyromania	64
Trichotillomania	65

Reel to Real: Psychiatric Conditions in Cinema

11. Personality Disorders
Paranoid Personality Disorder	66
Schizoid Personality Disorder	67
Schizotypal Personality Disorder	68
Antisocial Personality Disorder	69
Borderline Personality Disorder	70
Histrionic Personality Disorder	71
Narcissistic Personality Disorder	72
Avoidant Personality Disorder	73
Dependent Personality Disorder	74
Obsessive-Compulsive Personality Disorder	75

12. Disorders Usually First Diagnosed in Infancy, Childhood or Adolescence
Mild Mental Retardation	76
Moderate Mental Retardation	77
Reading Disorder	78
Phonological Disorder	79
Stuttering	80
Austistic Disorder	81
Asperger's Disorder	82
Attention-Deficit Hyperactivity Disorder	83
Conduct Disorder: Childhood-Onset Type	84
Conduct Disorder: Adolescent-Onset Type	85
Pica	86
Tourette's Disorder	87
Enuresis	88
Encopresis	89
Selective Mutism	90

13. Cognitive Disorders
Delirium	91
Dementia of the Alzheimer's Type	92
Dementia Due to Parkinson's Disease	93
Amnestic Disorder	94

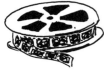

Table of Contents

14. Substance-Related Disorders

Alcohol Dependence	95
Alcohol Intoxication and Alcohol Withdrawal	96
Alcohol Withdrawal Delirium	97
Amphetamine Intoxication with Perceptual Disturbances	98
Caffeine Intoxication	99
Cannabis Abuse	100
Cocaine Abuse	101
Cocaine Intoxication	102
Hallucinogen Intoxication	103
Inhalant Intoxication	104
Nicotine Withdrawal	105
Opioid Intoxication	106
Opioid Dependence	107
Opioid Abuse	108
Sedative, Hypnotic or Anxiolytic Dependence	109
Sedative, Hypnotic or Anxiolytic Withdrawal	110

15. Mental Disorders Due to Medical Conditions

Psychotic Disorder Due to a Head Injury	111
Dementia Due to a Metabolic Abnormality	112
Amnestic Disorder and Personality Change Due to Anoxia	113
Mood Disorder Due to Porphyria	114
Mood Disorder Due to Corticosteroids	115
Catatonic Disorder Due to Encephalitis	116

Movie Index	117
All-Star Movie Recommendations	122
References	126
About the Author and Artist	128

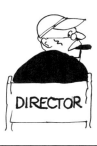

Reel to Real: Psychiatric Conditions in Cinema

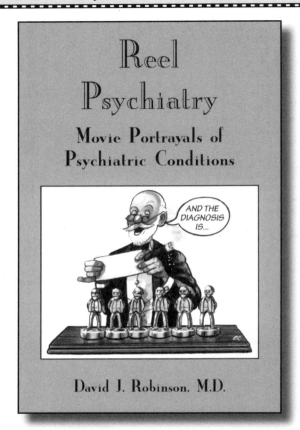

Reel to Real is condensed from:
Reel Psychiatry: Movie Portrayals of Psychiatric Conditions
ISBN: (13) 978-1-894328-07-4, (10) 1-894328-07-8
Soft Cover, 340 pages, 5½ x 8½ inches trim size
© Rapid Psychler Press, 2003

Differences from *Reel Psychiatry*

Reel to Real differs from *Reel Psychiatry* in the following ways:

- *Reel Psychiatry* has a section for each disorder called **Understanding the Condition**, where each diagnosis is clearly explained to give readers an overview of what is involved. Additionally, a section for each disorder called **Making the Diagnosis** that summarizes the diagnostic criteria from the DSM-IV-TR is included. Both of these features were not included in *Reel to Real* due to space limitations.

- *Reel Psychiatry* includes more movie listings, and in some chapters discusses individual symptoms in significant detail.

- *Reel Psychiatry* includes a rating system (fair, good, excellent) for the accuracy of the movie portrayals compared to what the condition is like in actual patients. *Reel to Real* includes, wherever possible, only the excellent portrayals. In some of the less accurate movie depictions however, there are often characters who display particular symptoms (but not the entire condition) or are seen too briefly to qualify for the diagnosis, but the movie contains segments that are of excellent quality for educational purposes.

- In *Reel Psychiatry*, there are extra sections explaining some interesting aspect of the group of conditions being presented. For example, the section in the Mood Disorders chapter features Creativity and Bipolar Disorder, and the chapter on Sleep Disorders contains information on the stages of human sleep. Due to space limitations, these sections were not included in *Reel to Real*.

- *Reel Psychiatry* contains a three-page chapter detailing the many similarities shared between cinema and the practice of psychiatry. Additionally, a seven-page chapter is included providing an overview of the diagnostic processes used in modern psychiatry.

- A twenty-one page chapter lists contacts for national organizations and web sites for many psychiatric conditions. Listings for the U.S. and Canada are included.

Movie Rating System

★

A portrayal of limited accuracy. One or two features of the condition may be well demonstrated and discussed in the presentation that follows but the overall example is relatively weak.

★★

An overall good portrayal with many features being consistent with the actual condition.

★★★

An excellent portrayal. The depiction is particularly accurate and conveys a strong sense of what the condition is actually like.

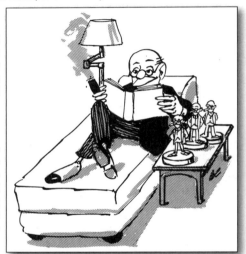

Disclaimers
Disclaimer #1

In *Reel to Real*, I have offered opinions on how accurately the character's role depicts an actual psychiatric illness. In the films that are portrayals of true stories, I am clearly NOT offering an opinion on the real person's condition. I haven't done any supplemental reading, nor reviewed any case reports, and have not interviewed any of the people whose lives are depicted in the movies listed in this book. Because of the artistic license

Rating System and Disclaimers

taken by film makers, I ask you to please keep in mind that someone may be affected by a very different illness than the one depicted in a film, or indeed, may not suffer from any illness at all.

Disclaimer #2
For ease of identification, the name of the actor is listed along with the name of the movie character. Again, I am offering an opinion on how close the portrayal is to a "real" patient. I am not giving an opinion on the quality of the performance. Many excellent films have fascinating characters that unfortunately are not suitable for the purposes of this book. In some cases it is the minor characters who provide accurate (but also often brief) portrayals. For some psychiatric conditions I have reviewed less popular films although I have tried to discuss movies that are easily accessible for rental or purchase. I am also most assuredly not making any comments about the actors' personal lives.

Disclaimer #3
Knowledge of the material in this book will not provide the reader with a sufficient enough basis for making psychiatric diagnoses. Mental health professionals spend years training to be able to distinguish the signs and symptoms of psychiatric illnesses and to be able to coalesce these findings into an accurate diagnosis. *Reel to Real* offers no shortcut to this process. Anyone professing expertise based solely from the material in this book is doing themselves, as well as the person being offered the opinion, a great disservice. I consider it akin to reading a book about swimming and then trying to swim across a lake (and then drowning).

Disclaimer #4
This book concerns itself primarily with diagnosis. I have largely avoided discussing the suspected origins of mental illness and how these conditions are treated. Where I have included such information, it should be considered to be of a general nature and not necessarily pertinent to the character being discussed. In some cases information about etiology was included to enhance the presentation of the material from the movie.

Reel to Real: **Psychiatric Conditions in Cinema**

Disclaimer #5
I completed a reasonable but not exhaustive survey of films in order to produce *Reel to Real*. I am certain that I have missed excellent portrayals from a wide variety of films. I encourage readers to contact me to share their knowledge of films that I have not listed here (I can be reached via rapid@psychler.com).

Disclaimer #6
I am not a world-renowned diagnostician. Certainly, a fertile discussion could ensue from any of the movies presented in this book and would generate a lengthy list of possible diagnoses. For the purposes of clarity and brevity, I have chosen to focus on what appears to me to be the principal diagnosis, and then note features that are less commonly seen or are inconsistent. I have not listed each possible condition that may apply to a certain cinematic portrayal.

Disclaimer #7
Movie makers have not been assigned the task of providing accurate depictions of every psychiatric condition. In some cases it was not possible to find portrayals of a certain illness. In other cases characters are amalgamations of many symptoms that do not lend themselves to a single, coherent diagnosis. Where necessary, specific aspects of a portrayal or certain scenes consistent with a diagnosis are presented, though the character's overall portrayal may not be that accurate a depiction.

Disclaimer #8
It has not been possible to include depictions of all the conditions or diagnostic categories listed in the DSM-IV-TR. Some are possibly too specific or too obscure to be worked into a movie plot.

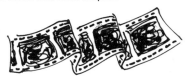

Disclaimers

Disclaimer #9
I am not a film critic nor a gossip columnist, though it was tempting at times to add some commentary to this effect. I haven't selected the movies presented in *Reel to Real* because they won awards, didn't win awards, featured a certain actor or were particularly notable for some reason. I have listed films that I believe have educational merit for readers interested in psychiatry. In the very few instances where I thought that viewers might be offended at the film's content, I have made comments to bring this to their attention.

Disclaimer #10
I have no financial connection to any studio, actor, video rental outlet, or other commercial source from which tapes or DVDs might be obtained. I recognize that the listing of a movie in this book may well lead to a number of people renting or purchasing the title. I am pleased with the prospect of the creative people who produced these movies benefiting from their hard work.

Disclaimer #11
All of the movies listed in this book are property of their respective studios, agencies, distribution companies, etc. Instructors who wish to use film clips in teaching situations are required to contact the proper representatives to obtain their permission.

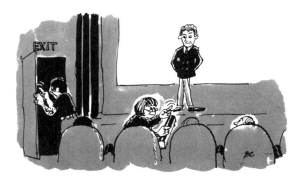

Reel to Real: Psychiatric Conditions in Cinema

Format Used in *Reel to Real*

 ## Movie Title

 Diagnosis Portrayed: Using DSM-IV-TR terminology
DSM-IV-TR Code: Precise coding from DSM-IV-TR

 Accuracy Rating:
★/★★★ (limited accuracy)   ★★/★★★ (good)
★★★/★★★ (excellent)

 Character's Name: Character with the condition
Actor's Name: Included for ease of identification

 Signs & Symptoms: The most prominent signs and symptoms are list in alphabetical order in this section. In some cases there are signs and symptoms that are unrelated to the main condition being portrayed by the character listed above. When this occurs, the diagnosis most often associated with the sign or symptom is indicated next to it.

 Year of Release: **Country:**
Language: *   **Genre:**   **Time:**
Information on the above features of the films has been included on the recommendation of many readers and reviewers of *Reel Psychiatry*. *Films not originally done in English are available in versions with subtitles.

PostScript:
This is additional commentary provided on the film, characters or diagnosis. In some instances reference is made to suspected etiology and on occasion some mention is made of a particular form of treatment for the condition being presented.

Psychotic Disorders

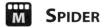 SPIDER

Diagnosis Portrayed: Schizophrenia, Disorganized Type
DSM-IV-TR Code: 295.10

Accuracy Rating:
★★★/★★★

Character's Name: Spider
Actor's Name: Ralph Fiennes

Signs & Symptoms:
Negative symptoms:
- Affective flattening
- Alogia
- Anhedonia
- Apathy
- Asociality
- Attention deficits
- Avolition

Speech abnormalities

Year of Release: 2002 **Country:** Canada/France/UK
Language: English **Genre:** Drama **Time:** 98 min.

PostScript:
Spider has schizophrenia marked by severe deficit symptoms (also called negative symptoms). He is released from an institution after many years and tries to re-establish himself at a boarding home. However, he either never developed many interests or social skills or lost them during his institutional stay. Soon after his release, he begins to regress and gets caught in a web of childhood memories causing him to misinterpret the world around him and to misidentify people as being significant from his past. The portrayal is remarkable because Spider rarely says anything discernible and mumbles the little dialogue that he has. He develops his own written language consisting of letter forms and other shapes.

Reel to Real: **Psychiatric Conditions in Cinema**

POSSESSED

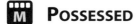

Diagnosis Portrayed: Schizophrenia, Catatonic Type
DSM-IV-TR Code: 295.20

Accuracy Rating:
★★★/★★★

Character's Name: Louise Howell
Actor's Name: Joan Crawford

Signs & Symptoms:
Catatonic symptoms:
- Catalepsy
- Echolalia
- Stupor
- Waxy flexibility

Delusions: erotomanic
Hallucinations: auditory
Overvalued ideas
Thought blocking

Year of Release: 1947 **Country:** USA
Language: English **Genre:** Drama **Time:** 108 min.

PostScript:
Joan Crawford starred in another film by this name in 1931. There are many good examples of psychopathology in this film. In the opening sequence, Louise is seen wandering in a disorganized state misidentifying every man she sees as "David." She lapses into a catatonic stupor and is taken to hospital. Once there, she is quickly identified as a psychiatric patient and given a further assessment. The conversation that ensues between the two examining physicians is accurate both in terms of their observations and use of psychiatric terminology. After receiving an injection in the emergency department, Louise has the auditory hallucination of a piano playing a piece composed by Schumann.

Psychotic Disorders

CANVAS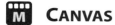

Diagnosis Portrayed: Schizophrenia, Paranoid Type
DSM-IV-TR Code: 295.30

Accuracy Rating:
★★★/★★★

Character's Name: Mary Marino
Actor's Name: Marcia Gay Harden

Signs & Symptoms:
Delusions:
 - Paranoid/persecutory
Derealization
Hallucinations:
 - Auditory

Year of Release: 2006 **Country:** USA
Language: English **Genre:** Drama **Time:** 101 min.

PostScript:
Canvas is an accurate and sympathetic portrayal of Mary, a woman with schizophrenia and the effects that her illness has on her son and husband. Mary has some quirks at the beginning of the film, but then decompensates quickly into a state of agitation and paranoia and requires an involuntary hospitalization after being taken from her home by the police. Situations common to many serious mental illness are shown, including Mary's husband John (Joe Pantoliano) arguing with their insurance company for coverage, and Mary repeatedly denying that she has an illness or needs medication. *Canvas* received praise from both professionals and patients for its sensitive handling of psychotic symptoms and the family's adjustments, which are significant and continuous. The film is rich in recurring symbols and imagery, with the title being expressed in at least three themes. In contrast to *Spider* or *Clean, Shaven*, this movie has a much more optimistic ending.

Reel to Real: Psychiatric Conditions in Cinema

CLEAN, SHAVEN

Diagnosis Portrayed: Schizophrenia, Undifferentiated Type
DSM-IV-TR Code: 295.90

Accuracy Rating:
★★★ / ★★★

Character's Name: Peter Winter
Actor's Name: Peter Greene

Signs & Symptoms:
Delusions:
- Paranoid/persecutory
- Somatic

Hallucinations:
- Auditory
- Command

Negative symptoms:
- Affective flattening
- Alogia

Year of Release: 1993 **Country:** USA
Language: English **Genre:** Drama **Time:** 79 min.

PostScript:
Winter leaves a mental institution to search for his daughter, who was long ago given up for adoption. He suffers from psychotic symptoms for most of the film, and at times has vivid hallucinatory experiences that leave the viewer wondering what actually transpired. Winter believes that he had surgery while in the psychiatric hospital and had a transmitter embedded in his finger and a receiver somewhere in his head. These somatic delusions help explain Winter's self-mutilation — cutting his scalp and excising a fingernail. He is so disconnected from reality at these times that he doesn't feel any pain. He removes most of his body hair, but no explanation is given for why he does this.

Psychotic Disorders

 # BELL JAR, THE

 Diagnosis Portrayed: Schizophreniform Disorder
DSM-IV-TR Code: 295.40

 Accuracy Rating:
★★★/★★★

 Character's Name: Esther Greenwood
Actor's Name: Marilyn Hassett

 Signs & Symptoms: Acute phase of psychosis
Negative symptoms:
- Asociality

Prodromal phase of psychosis

 Year of Release: 1979 **Country:** USA
Language: English **Genre:** Drama **Time:** 107 min.

PostScript:
This film is based on the book by Sylvia Plath. Esther is a straight-A college junior who wins a poetry award, and later, a chance to write for a women's magazine in New York for a summer. Prior to leaving, two scenes could be considered as being consistent with a psychotic prodrome: her oddly emotionless probing into her father's death, and her marked ambivalence about many things, including her boyfriend's offer of marriage. In the acute phase of her illness (in her mother's house), we see Esther in a regressed state, showing negative symptoms, particularly social withdrawal and poor hygiene. The time course and severity of symptoms favor schizophreniform disorder over schizophrenia. A rough calculation is that Esther was hospitalized two weeks after her return from New York and started to make a recovery about two months later. The total time course appears to be less than six months. Esther also appears to make a full recovery, which happens less frequently with schizophrenia, but is more typical of other psychotic disorders.

Reel to Real: Psychiatric Conditions in Cinema

SHINE

Diagnosis Portrayed: Schizoaffective Disorder
DSM-IV-TR Code: 295.70

Accuracy Rating:
★★★/★★★

Character's Name: David Helfgott
Actor's Name: Geoffrey Rush

Signs & Symptoms:
Mood changes: elation
Negative symptoms
Residual phase of psychosis
Thought process abnormalities:
- Derailment
- Flight of ideas
- Incoherence
- Loosening of associations

Year of Release: 1996 **Country:** Australia
Language: English **Genre:** Drama **Time:** 105 min.

PostScript:
The character of David provides a good demonstration of thought derailment, and at times, incoherence. The opening scene contains a monologue with the central theme of a cat, but is otherwise extremely difficult to follow. As an adult (the scenes played by Geoffrey Rush), David demonstrates a persistently jovial mood, seeking hugs from everyone, and is rather disinhibited regarding where his hands travel around women that he fancies. His speech pattern is unusual and at times lacks clear connections between ideas. On other occasions it contains puns and references that are off topic but can be understood as being related to a central theme. These features make the condition portrayed in *Shine* consistent with schizoaffective disorder.

Psychotic Disorders

 # He Loves Me... He Loves Me Not

 Diagnosis Portrayed: Delusional Disorder: Erotomanic
DSM-IV-TR Code: 297.1

 Accuracy Rating:
★★★/★★★

 Character's Name: Angélique
Actor's Name: Audrey Tautou

 Signs & Symptoms: Delusions: erotomanic
Non-bizarre delusions

 Year of Release: 2002 **Country:** France
Language: French   **Genre:** Thriller   **Time:** 92 min.

PostScript:
Erotomania (also called *delusional loving*, *phantom lover syndrome*, and *Clérambault's complex*) is beautifully portrayed in this French film staring Audrey Tautou as Angélique, a young art student ostensibly having an affair with a married cardiologist, Loic (Samuel Le Bihan). The movie is first told from her perspective, where we see them interact with each other and events appear to be progressing to the point where they will take a vacation together and Loic may leave his pregnant wife. Angélique's friends try to persuade her to come to her senses, but she is smitten and hopes beyond hope, clinging to small gestures and then dismissing anything that seems to contradict her wishes. In a masterful piece of filmmaking, we are then able to see events as they actually occurred (not simply Loic's version). Angélique misinterprets a whimsical gesture from Loic and then begins to pursue him and resorts to increasingly dramatic and dangerous behaviors to get his attention. Angélique attempts suicide, and later commits murder when her love for Loic is unrequited. She is hospitalized for some period of time, making a collage out of the pills that she was prescribed but never took.

Reel to Real: Psychiatric Conditions in Cinema

SNAKE PIT, THE

Diagnosis Portrayed: Delusional Disorder: Grandiose
DSM-IV-TR Code: 297.1

Accuracy Rating:
★★★/★★★

Character's Name: Inmate Countess
Actor's Name: Grayce Hampton

Signs & Symptoms: Delusions: grandiose
Non-bizarre delusions

Year of Release: 1948 **Country:** USA
Language: English **Genre:** Thriller **Time:** 108 min.

PostScript:
An illustration of grandiose delusions is presented on Ward 1 by the woman with the lace gloves. She mentions that her husband is very wealthy and owns the Hope Diamond. When Virginia (Olivia de Havilland) teases her by saying that she owns the "Hopeless Emerald," the woman misses the pun and belittles the (fictitious) gem as having a flaw, making it unsuitable for her beautiful hands. This woman misunderstands Virginia's use of the word "general." Toying with her further, Virginia changes the statement about the "general you" to "General Pershing," whom the delusional woman immediately names as a member of a "minor branch" of her family.

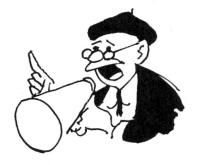

Psychotic Disorders

 # UNFAITHFULLY YOURS

 Diagnosis Portrayed: Delusional Disorder: Infidelity
DSM-IV-TR Code: 297.1

 Accuracy Rating:
★★★/★★★

 Character's Name: Claude Eastman
Actor's Name: Dudley Moore

 Signs & Symptoms: Delusions: infidelity/jealousy
Non-bizarre delusions

Year of Release: 1984 **Country:** USA
Language: English **Genre:** Comedy **Time:** 96 min.

PostScript:
This is a remake of the 1948 film starring Rex Harrison and Linda Darnell in the lead roles. Eastman is a famous orchestra conductor who has recently married the vivacious and much younger Daniella (Nastassja Kinski), an Italian actress. Prior to leaving on a tour, Claude asks his butler to keep an "eye" on Daniella, but instead a "private eye" is hired. Claude, wary of their age difference, cannot help but watch the video surveillance tape taken by the detective, which shows a man visiting their apartment late at night. Eastman learns that this was Max (Armand Assante), a close friend. Everywhere Eastman turns, more circumstantial evidence accumulates to support his fear that Max and Daniella are lovers (Max is having an affair, but not with Daniella). When Claude confronts Max a heated argument ensues but because of their mutual vagueness, Claude's indignation reaches a fever pitch (with predictably humorous results). In severe cases of delusional infidelity, the affected person might report that his or her partner has dozens of encounters over the span of a day. It can become so extreme that any brief absence from the person's direct view will result in a torrent of accusations.

Reel to Real: **Psychiatric Conditions in Cinema**

UNSTRUNG HEROES

Diagnosis Portrayed: Delusional Disorder: Persecutory
DSM-IV-TR Code: 297.1

Accuracy Rating:
★★★ / ★★★

Character's Name: Michael Richards
Actor's Name: Danny Lidz

Signs & Symptoms: Delusions: paranoid/persecutory
Non-bizarre delusions

Year of Release: 1995   **Country:** USA
Language: English   **Genre:** Drama   **Time:** 93 min.

PostScript:
Lidz is an uncle to the main character in this movie. He literally explodes onto the scene at the family gathering where we first meet him. Danny's brother opens a window for him to crawl through, because he (presumably) wanted to avoid detection. Danny immediately pulls the blinds down and closes the door that connects to the patio. He insists that there were two men following him, but through a series of sly maneuvers he was able to elude them. He then espouses his belief that everyone in the room is being monitored and talks into one woman's necklace because he thinks she has a microphone hidden there. He accuses his sister-in-law Selma (Andie McDowell) of smoking marijuana, which is untrue. Danny goes on to dominate the gathering with his persecutory beliefs, such as Eisenhower being a Nazi. Meanwhile, he tells Selma that she looks like death and that she should get some air (she is in fact dying of cancer at this time). Later in the film, Danny accuses a seventh grade student of being a fascist and believes that life is made up of anti-Semitic conspiracies. He also believes there are only eight trustworthy people in the world, though he doesn't disclose who he thinks they are. . .

Psychotic Disorders

Bug

Diagnosis Portrayed: Delusional Disorder: Somatic
DSM-IV-TR Code: 297.1

Accuracy Rating:
★★★/★★★

Character's Name: Peter Evans
Actor's Name: Michael Shannon

Signs & Symptoms:
Delusion: formication
Delusion: somatic
Shared psychotic disorder

Year of Release: 2006 **Country:** USA
Language: English **Genre:** Thriller **Time:** 102 min.

PostScript:
Agnes (Ashley Judd) is a lonely waitress who lives in a rundown Oklahoma motel. Her abusive ex-husband Jerry Goss (Harry Connick, Jr.) is due to be released from state prison and she is worried that he'll seek her out. Agnes' one friend R.C. (Lynn Collins) introduces her to Evans, a peculiar, paranoiac drifter and they stumble into a romantic relationship. However, as Evans grows more comfortable with Agnes he begins to reveal secrets about his past and preoccupation with being infested with microscopic organisms.

Evans believes that he finds bugs in their bed, and discloses that he was a soldier in the Gulf War and was involuntarily subjected to experiments by the army. He grows more frantic in his quest to have Agnes agree with him, and in doing so engages in inducing a shared psychotic disorder (folie à deux) in Agnes. She is rendered vulnerable to Evan's delusions because of her desire to maintain their relationship, but also due to her isolation, fear of Goss, and the distant disappearance of her son, from which she has never recovered.

Reel to Real: Psychiatric Conditions in Cinema

 ## HEAVENLY CREATURES

 Diagnosis Portrayed: Shared Psychotic Disorder
DSM-IV-TR Code: 297.3

 Accuracy Rating:
★★/★★★

 Character's Names: Pauline Rieper/Juliet Hulme
Actor's Name: Melanie Lynskey/Kate Winslet

 Signs & Symptoms: Folie à deux
Induced psychotic disorder

 Year of Release: 1994 **Country:** New Zealand/UK
Language: English **Genre:** Crime **Time:** 99 min.

PostScript:
This is a true story involving Pauline, a sullen teenager who befriends Juliet, who is fanciful and artistically gifted. Juliet speaks of a "fourth world" — her version of heaven — replete with music and art. This vision is shared between the two as a medieval fantasy, initially a romance but with a flavor of brutality. They escape into this kingdom via a gateway in the clouds that they believe to be open only two days per year. They consider themselves to be unappreciated creative geniuses. Immersing themselves in this fantasy world they assume the lead roles and construct elaborate tales that they hope to publish. Each dissociates into this world during difficult times and fantasizes that the kingdom's murderous heir disposes of those who would dare upset them. Eventually, they scheme to do away with Pauline's mother, who opposes their leaving New Zealand. This film is a good example of how a folie à deux starts and progresses, but falls short because the mother is killed for reasons unrelated to the girls' delusions. If the mother had been incorporated into the fantasy world as someone who threatened their relationship (e.g. as an evil witch) the portrayal would be more precise.

Mood Disorders

 WRONG MAN, THE

 Diagnosis Portrayed: Major Depressive Disorder, Single Episode, Severe With Psychotic Features
DSM-IV-TR Code: 296.24

 Accuracy Rating:
★★★/★★★

 Character's Name: Rose Balastrero
Actor's Name: Vera Miles

 Signs & Symptoms:
Anhedonia
Depressed mood
Diminished appetite
Diminished concentration
Feelings of guilt and worthlessness
Mood-congruent psychotic features
Psychomotor retardation and agitation

 Year of Release: 1956 **Country:** USA
Language: English **Genre:** Drama **Time:** 105 min.

PostScript:
Rose is the wife of a man wrongly accused of armed robbery. Her impacted wisdom teeth require treatment, and to pay the dentist, her husband borrows against an insurance policy. When he is at the insurance office, the clerk believes that he is the guilty party and calls the police. As their financial situation worsens and her husband's case looks progressively bleaker, Rose develops marked symptoms of depression. She believes that it is pointless to care about the outcome of the trial because everything is fixed against them. Rose launches into a tirade of delusional accusations and denouncements. She intends to keep her family at home, and will lock the doors to keep "them" out.

Reel to Real: Psychiatric Conditions in Cinema

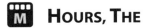
HOURS, THE

Diagnosis Portrayed: Major Depressive Disorder, Recurrent, Severe Without Psychotic Features
DSM-IV-TR Code: 296.33

Accuracy Rating:
★★★/★★★

Character's Name: Virginia Woolf
Actor's Name: Nicole Kidman

Character's Name: Laura Brown
Actor's Name: Julianne Moore

Character's Name: Richard Brown
Actor's Name: Ed Harris

Signs & Symptoms: Depressed mood
Suicidality

Year of Release: 2002 **Country:** USA/UK
Language: English **Genre:** Drama **Time:** 114 min.

PostScript:
The Hours teems with depressive themes and characters. The opening sequence features Virginia Woolf leaving a final note for her husband and then drowning herself, giving an outstanding glimpse into an articulate mind seeing only bleakness and hopelessness. Laura Brown is a depressed mother/wife in the 1950's who seemingly has a perfect life. She plans to overdose, but then changes her mind and instead lives a hollow life. Richard Brown, her adoring son, becomes a successful writer who contracts AIDS and decides to take his life by jumping out of a window just prior to an event being planned in his honor.

Mood Disorders

 ## Patch Adams

Diagnosis Portrayed: Major Depressive Disorder, Single Episode, Moderate
DSM-IV-TR Code: 296.22

Accuracy Rating:
★★★/★★★

Character's Name: Hunter "Patch" Adams
Actor's Name: Robin Williams

Signs & Symptoms:
Depressed mood
Feelings of guilt and worthlessness
Leaden paralysis (atypical depression)
Psychomotor retardation
Suicidal thoughts

Year of Release: 1998 **Country:** USA
Language: English **Genre:** Comedy **Time:** 115 min.

PostScript:
Adams describes his feelings of disconnectedness and inner torment by using the metaphor of walking in circles for days in a driving snowstorm. He feels as if his legs are heavy (leaden paralysis) and that his shouts disappear in the wind. As this is being narrated, Adams, unshaven and listless, stares vacantly out of a bus window and appears apathetic. Adams realizes that the storm is in his mind, and uses an eloquent quote from Dante to describe his state of depression, "*In the middle of the journey of my life, I found myself in a dark wood, for I had lost the right path.*" Adams is tempted to take an overdose, but instead admits himself into a psychiatric facility to seek help. Once at the hospital his face is expressionless. He walks slowly, looks bewildered, and is easily overwhelmed. Later, when he tells his personal history to his psychiatrist, Adams reveals that when he was nine years old he lost his father.

Reel to Real: Psychiatric Conditions in Cinema

M HOSPITAL, THE

Dx **Diagnosis Portrayed:** Dysthymic Disorder
DSM-IV-TR Code: 300.4

★ **Accuracy Rating:**
★★/★★★

C **Character's Name:** Dr. Herbert Bock
Actor's Name: George C. Scott

Sx **Signs & Symptoms:**
Concentration is impaired
Depressed mood for at least 2 years
Energy level is decreased
Hopelessness
Self-esteem is diminished
Suicidal thoughts

I **Year of Release:** 1971 **Country:** USA
Language: English **Genre:** Drama **Time:** 103 min.

PostScript:
Bock is a departmental chief in a major New York City hospital. His performance at work has noticeably declined. He dwells on suicide and has considered a method that will avoid detection so his family can still claim insurance benefits. While giving his life narrative, he admits to having felt depressed for a period of years, possibly extending back to college. He seems beaten down by his situation, and walks slowly with his head hanging down. Unfortunately (for this portrayal), Bock uses alcohol heavily throughout the movie. This complicates his situation, and in fact he almost attempts suicide when he is drunk in his office. His mental abilities are difficult to gauge, though in one scene he confides to a medical student that he's glad that they are discussing tuberculosis because that was the only condition he read about before giving the teaching session.

Mood Disorders

 # Mosquito Coast, The

 Diagnosis Portrayed: Bipolar I Disorder, Most Recent Episode Manic, Severe With Mood-Incongruent Psychotic Features
DSM-IV-TR Code: 296.44

 Accuracy Rating:
★★/★★★

 Character's Name: Allie Fox
Actor's Name: Harrison Ford

 Signs & Symptoms:
Dangerous activities
Decreased need for sleep
Grandiosity
Increase in goal-directed activity
Paranoia (psychotic symptom)
Pressured speech

 Year of Release: 1986 **Country:** USA
Language: English **Genre:** Drama **Time:** 117 min.

PostScript:
Allie abruptly quits his job as a laborer and decides an instant later to travel to Central America to build a self-sustaining refrigerator for the native population. Rather than just being rebellious or strongly individualistic, Allie demonstrates many symptoms of mania with mood-incongruent psychotic features in this film, including: setting fire to a chapel; wanting to go further into a jungle with his wife and young children (but without food, possessions, or fuel); baseless accusations of his wife not supporting him; and denying his need for medical attention after being shot. His mood at the beginning of the film is expansive and charming, but it becomes progressively more and more irritable.

Reel to Real: Psychiatric Conditions in Cinema

Mr. Jones

Diagnosis Portrayed: Bipolar I Disorder, Most Recent Episode Manic, Severe Without Psychotic Features
DSM-IV-TR Code: 296.43

Accuracy Rating:
★★★/★★★

Character's Name: Mr. Jones/Amanda Chang
Actor's Name: Richard Gere/Lauren Tom

Signs & Symptoms:
Distractibility
Flight of ideas
Grandiosity
Increase in goal-directed activity
Pleasurable activities that have a high potential for painful consequences
Pressured speech

Year of Release: 1993 **Country:** USA
Language: English **Genre:** Drama **Time:** 114 min.

PostScript:
Mr. Jones rides his bike to a construction site and charms the foreman into letting him work there. Claiming he can do the work of two men, Jones will work the first day free of charge but expects to be paid double the next day and predicts he'll have the foreman's job by the third. Jones is too distractible to work efficiently, getting carried away by the constant air traffic near the construction site. He soon begins to think that he can fly, necessitating hospitalization on an involuntary basis. Once at the hospital, Jones' treating psychiatrist also cares for a female patient named Amanda, who gives an excellent portrayal of pressured speech in the scene where she describes how she got her name.

Mood Disorders

MICHAEL CLAYTON

Diagnosis Portrayed: Bipolar I Disorder, Most Recent Episode Manic, Moderate
DSM-IV-TR Code: 296.42

Accuracy Rating:
★★★/★★★

Character's Name: Arthur Edens
Actor's Name: Tom Wilkinson

Signs & Symptoms:
Distractibility
Flight of ideas
Increase in goal-directed activity
Pleasurable activities that have a high potential for painful consequences
Pressured speech

Year of Release: 2007 **Country:** USA
Language: English **Genre:** Crime **Time:** 119 min.

PostScript:
Edens is a successful litigator who represents a chemical company that suppressed information about the toxicity of one of their insecticides. He has a history of bipolar disorder that has responded well to previous treatment. In the course of preparing for the examination for discovery, Eden's mood escalates and he unilaterally decides he can no longer defend his guilty client. As if to shed a patina of denial regarding his role in preparing their defense, Edens disrobes in front of everyone at the discovery as well as the video camera recording the event. Edens then goes on to explain his motivation to the law firm's fixer, Michael Clayton (George Clooney). While Eden's actions may superficially appear commendable, he violates his attorney-client agreement and could have chosen a less destructive way of being taken off the case.

Reel to Real: Psychiatric Conditions in Cinema

MAD LOVE

Diagnosis Portrayed: Cyclothymic Disorder
DSM-IV-TR Code: 301.13

Accuracy Rating:
★★★/★★★

Character's Name: Casey Roberts
Actor's Name: Drew Barrymore

Signs & Symptoms:
Depressive symptoms:
- Depressed mood
- Diminished ability to concentrate
- Psychomotor agitation
- Thoughts of suicide

Hypomanic symptoms:
- Distractibility
- Inflated self-esteem
- Increase in goal-directed activity
- Pleasurable activities that have a high potential for painful consequences

Year of Release: 1995 **Country:** USA
Language: English **Genre:** Drama **Time:** 93 min.

PostScript:
Casey exhibits significant mood lability in this film, ranging from being despondent and taking an overdose to displaying grandiosity and recklessness. Her mood changes do not last long enough, are not severe enough, and change too quickly for her to qualify for the diagnosis of bipolar disorder. Casey is rarely without significant mood symptoms in the film. She seems to have had this mood lability for an extended period of time based on the additional information given by her parents.

Anxiety Disorders

 ## ANALYZE THIS

 Diagnosis Portrayed: Panic Disorder
Without Agoraphobia
DSM-IV-TR Code: 300.01

 Accuracy Rating:
★★★/★★★

 Character's Name: Paul Vitti
Actor's Name: Robert De Niro

 Signs & Symptoms:
Changes in behavior due to the attacks
Chest pains
Choking sensation
Dizziness
Fear of dying
Persistent concerns of having more panic attacks
Shortness of breath
Sweating
Worry about the consequences of the panic attacks

 Year of Release: 1999 **Country:** USA/Australia
Language: English **Genre:** Comedy **Time:** 103 min.

PostScript:
The murder of one of Vitti's father's friends causes Paul to experience repeated panic attacks. In one scene, he becomes abruptly uneasy and restless, fearing that he is having a heart attack. Speeding to the ER, he is told that he has had a "panic attack" and immediately assaults the doctor for suggesting that anyone in Vitti's line of work would actually panic. Vitti seeks treatment from Dr. Ben Sobel (Billy Crystal), who isn't initially sure how to help his distressed patient.

Reel to Real: Psychiatric Conditions in Cinema

COPYCAT

Diagnosis Portrayed: Agoraphobia Without History of Panic Disorder
DSM-IV-TR Code: 300.22

Accuracy Rating:
★★★/★★★

Character's Name: Helen Hudson
Actor's Name: Sigourney Weaver

Signs & Symptoms: Anxiety about being in places or situations from which escape might be difficult or in which help may not be available
Situations are avoided or endured with marked distress

Year of Release: 1995 **Country:** USA
Language: English **Genre:** Crime **Time:** 123 min.

PostScript:
Helen is a mental health professional who has made a career out of studying serial killers. Her testimony helped convict Daryll Lee Cullum (Harry Connick, Jr.), ostensibly because she proved that he did not suffer from a mental illness. Cullum subsequently escaped and viciously attacked her, but was re-arrested. Helen went on to suffer from severe anxiety symptoms and became housebound. The extent of her agoraphobia is very well demonstrated in a scene where she must retrieve a newspaper. It has been dropped in the apartment hallway just out of arm's reach. When Helen can't reach it with a broom, she becomes highly distressed just walking a couple of feet outside to pick it up. Later in the film, Helen chooses to stay in her apartment even when an intruder is there, since venturing outside is even more terrifying to her.

Anxiety Disorders

In Country

Diagnosis Portrayed: Posttraumatic Stress Disorder
DSM-IV-TR Code: 309.81

Accuracy Rating:
★★★ / ★★★

Character's Name: Emmett Smith
Actor's Name: Bruce Willis

Signs & Symptoms:
Avoiding thoughts, feelings, or conversations associated with the event
Difficulty falling or staying asleep
Exaggerated startle response
Feeling detached/estranged
Intense distress upon exposure to anything reminiscent of the event
Irritability/outbursts of anger
Markedly diminished interest in significant activities
Restricted range of emotions

Year of Release: 1989 **Country:** USA
Language: English **Genre:** Drama **Time:** 120 min.

PostScript:
Emmett is a Vietnam veteran who lives with his niece Samantha (Emily Lloyd). At the beginning of the film, he is attending Samantha's graduation ceremony. The steely voice of the man giving the commencement address reminds him of an officer's farewell he listened to as he shipped out for Vietnam. Emmett experiences flashbacks of combat during a thunderstorm. At a dance arranged to honor veterans, Anita, a nurse with an interest in Emmett, has difficulty getting him to dance with her due to his sense of estrangement from others.

Reel to Real: Psychiatric Conditions in Cinema

 # MATCHSTICK MEN

 Diagnosis Portrayed: Obsessive-Compulsive Disorder
DSM-IV-TR Code: 300.3

 Accuracy Rating:
★★★/★★★

 Character's Name: Roy Waller
Actor's Name: Nicholas Cage

 Signs & Symptoms:
Obsessions:
- Contamination
- Order/symmetry
- Safety

Compulsions:
- Checking
- Cleaning
- Counting
- Eating

 Year of Release: 2003 **Country:** USA
Language: English **Genre:** Comedy **Time:** 116 min.

PostScript:
Roy is a con artist who prides himself on his ability to get people to give him their money instead of him taking it. He runs clever scams with his partner Frank (Sam Rockwell). Roy is an anxious man most of the time, but when his medication runs out his OCD symptoms worsen, effectively disabling him. He opens and closes doors three times while counting out loud in foreign languages. He cleans his house meticulously as a means of reducing his obsessions about dirt and contamination. He likes rituals and order, and has a very restricted diet (mainly tuna) unless he has a need to eat in more social circumstances. He also develops vocal and motor tics when stressed, but these are not typical for OCD.

Anxiety Disorders

Annie Hall

Diagnosis Portrayed: Generalized Anxiety Disorder
DSM-IV-TR Code: 300.02

Accuracy Rating:
★★★/★★★

Character's Name: Alvy Singer
Actor's Name: Woody Allen

Signs & Symptoms:
Anxiety is difficult to control
Difficulty concentrating
Excessive anxiety that occurs more days than not
Irritability

Year of Release: 1977 **Country:** USA
Language: English **Genre:** Comedy **Time:** 93 min.

PostScript:
Some of Alvy's multitudinous concerns are as follows:
- The possibility of a conspiracy in the JFK assassination so absorbs him that he can't be intimate with his first wife
- Everything that his parents told him was good (sun, milk, red meat, college) he deems to ultimately be bad for him
- He wants to kiss Annie early during their first date so that he will be less anxious and better able to digest his dinner
- He keeps a first aid kit, insect spray, and a fire alarm handy so that he can be prepared for emergencies
- He panders to the audience and passers-by to show that he is being maligned, and enlists their assistance in deciding what is "normal"
- He becomes defensive and irritable around accomplished people
- He pays for Annie's analysis, and then gets jealous because she makes progress at a faster rate than he does

Reel to Real: **Psychiatric Conditions in Cinema**

HIGH ANXIETY

Diagnosis Portrayed: Specific Phobia
DSM-IV-TR Code: 300.29

Accuracy Rating:
★★/★★★

Character's Name: Richard H. Thorndyke
Actor's Name: Mel Brooks

Signs & Symptoms: Exposure to the object or situation almost invariably provokes an immediate anxiety response
Marked and persistent fear that is unreasonable, excessive, and cued by the object or situation
The person recognizes that the fear is excessive or unreasonable

Year of Release: 1977 **Country:** USA
Language: English **Genre:** Comedy **Time:** 94 min.

PostScript:
This movie spoofs at least a half dozen of Alfred Hitchcock's films, though it focuses primarily on *Vertigo*. The title of this film is a pun referring to both the main character's general level of nervousness and his particular fear of heights. Thorndyke is a psychiatrist who becomes the administrator of the Psycho-Neurotic Institute for the Very, Very Nervous. Thorndyke's aversion to heights is evident throughout the movie because he is unable to avoid situations such as taking airplanes or riding in elevators. Even his office overlooks a sheer cliff face. Thorndyke develops clear symptoms of anxiety when exposed to heights, particularly when an old friend insists that he take in the panoramic view from his office by standing on the edge of a cliff.

Anxiety Disorders

 # DEFENDING YOUR LIFE

 Diagnosis Portrayed: Social Phobia
DSM-IV-TR Code: 300.23

 Accuracy Rating:
★★★/★★★

 Character's Name: Daniel Miller
Actor's Name: Albert Brooks

 Signs & Symptoms:
Being exposed to the feared social situation (e.g. public speaking) almost invariably provokes anxiety
Marked and persistent fears in social or performance situations where a person feels that he or she will do something that is humiliating or embarrassing, or will show anxiety
The fear is recognized as being unreasonable under the circumstances

 Year of Release: 1991 **Country:** USA
Language: English **Genre:** Comedy **Time:** 112 min.

PostScript:
Miller dies an untimely death and needs to undergo a review of his life by a panel of higher beings before his fate is decided upon. The panel, arranged much like a courtroom, looks at selected experiences from his life to decide if he lived his life fully and courageously and is deserving of going on to a more desirable place in the universe. There is a segment that reviews his mounting anxiety and desperation at a public speaking engagement. Miller will seemingly bargain away anything to be able to get out of the situation and becomes tremulous and sweaty before ultimately freezing in front of the crowd.

Reel to Real: Psychiatric Conditions in Cinema

HANNA AND HER SISTERS

Diagnosis Portrayed: Hypochondriasis
DSM-IV-TR Code: 300.7

Accuracy Rating:
★★★/★★★

Character's Name: Mickey Sachs
Actor's Name: Woody Allen

Signs & Symptoms:
Beliefs are not of delusional intensity and not limited only to appearance
Medical evaluation and reassurance do not lessen the preoccupation
Persistent fears of having a serious illness based on misinterpretation of minor bodily symptoms

Year of Release: 1986 **Country:** USA
Language: English **Genre:** Comedy **Time:** 103 min.

PostScript:
Mickey is the prototypic hypochondriac. Neurotic and plaintive, much of his role centers on his health concerns. A screen labeling him as a hypochondriac is shown before he even speaks. As Mickey is on the way to see his doctor he feels that this time (in contrast to other visits) he really has something that is slowly ruining his health. He had previously been concerned that his adenoids were causing problems for him, but withdrew this complaint when he was reminded that they'd already been removed. In another scene, a co-worker reminds him of the time that he thought he had a melanoma because he had a new spot on his back, but the spot was actually on his shirt. This portrayal is an excellent one because the viewer is party to Mickey's thoughts as he goes through the ordeal of not knowing if he has a serious illness (or not).

Somatoform Disorders

BANDITS

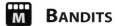

Diagnosis Portrayed: Conversion Disorder
DSM-IV-TR Code: 300.11

Accuracy Rating:
★★★/★★★

Character's Name: Terry Lee Collins
Actor's Name: Billy Bob Thornton

Signs & Symptoms:
Psychological factors are deemed to be associated with the onset of the symptom or deficit
Symptoms or deficits affecting voluntary movement or sensation suggest a neurological or medical condition
Symptoms or deficits are not being intentionally produced

Year of Release: 2001 **Country:** USA
Language: English **Genre:** Comedy **Time:** 123 min.

PostScript:
Collins states that his *"body chemistry is extraordinarily sensitive to suggestion and any symptom can be manufactured given the right circumstances, and that, by the way, doesn't mean that it isn't real."* In order to take revenge against Collins for attempting to steal his girlfriend, Blake (Bruce Willis) invents a story about a fictitious brother with a brain tumor. Blake says that his brother suffered from headaches, and as the symptoms became more pronounced, smelled burning feathers. This story strongly affects the suggestible Collins who, while in the middle of a bank robbery, asks an employee to check to see if his pupils are unequal. Shortly afterwards, Collins smells burning feathers and then develops numb lips and weakness on the right side of his body.

Reel to Real: Psychiatric Conditions in Cinema

RED DRAGON

Diagnosis Portrayed: Body Dysmorphic Disorder
DSM-IV-TR Code: 300.7

Accuracy Rating:
★★/★★★

Character's Name: Francis Dolarhyde
Actor's Name: Ralph Fiennes

Signs & Symptoms: Preoccupation with a slight or imagined defect in appearance

Year of Release: 2002 **Country:** USA/Germany
Language: English **Genre:** Thriller **Time:** 124 min.

PostScript:
Dolarhyde has a cleft lip that was surgically repaired, leaving him with a scar on his upper lip and a slight speech impediment. Although there is more affecting Dolarhyde than body dysmorphic disorder, he demonstrates many of the common characteristics of this condition. Dolarhyde is quite shy, and probably chose to work in a photographic laboratory because of the isolation it provides. Reba McClane (Emily Watson) is the only woman he feels comfortable with because she is blind. Even still, he doesn't like her touching his face and he doesn't respond favorably when she comments on his slight speech impediment. Dolarhyde engages in strenuous body building to compensate for (or distract himself and others from) his "defect." The mirrors in Dolarhyde's house are smashed, as are those in the homes where he commits violent crimes. He has a huge tattoo of a red dragon on his back, but it is unclear if this was done for the purpose of distraction or something else. What is missing from this portrayal is Dolarhyde's account of his symptoms, which are not revealed. Also, there is clearly a psychotic component to Dolarhyde's illness which is not typical for this condition.

Factitious Disorder

 ## DON'T SAY A WORD

 Diagnosis Portrayed: Factitious Disorder With Predominantly Psychological Signs and Symptoms
DSM-IV-TR Code: 300.16

 Accuracy Rating:
★/★★★

 Character's Name: Elisabeth Burroughs
Actor's Name: Brittany Murphy

 Signs & Symptoms: Intentional production or feigning of symptoms
The motivation for feigning symptoms is to assume the sick role

 Year of Release: 2001 **Country:** USA/Australia
Language: English **Genre:** Crime **Time:** 113 min.

PostScript:
Elisabeth saw her father, a bank robber, get brutally murdered in a subway station. For the next ten years she found ways to get admitted to psychiatric institutions by imitating almost 20 different diagnoses. Dr. Nathan Conrad (Michael Douglas) pieces together the inconsistencies from her medical record and recognizes that her catatonic symptoms (waxy flexibility) are not real. Elisabeth learned how to mimic a wide variety of psychiatric conditions, apparently for the purpose of staying in hospitals. Later in the film, this is shown to be a helpful strategy for Elisabeth because she is being pursued by her father's killers. This portrayal is less than ideal because Elisabeth clearly does have a reason for wanting to "assume the sick role" and would more accurately be diagnosed with malingering (see page 46). Also, Elisabeth has some symptoms of PTSD because of the trauma she experienced in seeing her father murdered.

Reel to Real: Psychiatric Conditions in Cinema

THE ROYAL TENENBAUMS

Diagnosis Portrayed: Malingering
DSM-IV-TR Code: V65.2

Accuracy Rating:
★★★/★★★

Character's Name: Royal Tenenbaum
Actor's Name: Gene Hackman

Signs & Symptoms: Conscious, intentional production of physical or psychological symptoms for the purpose of benefitting from an external incentive.

Year of Release: 2001 **Country:** USA
Language: English **Genre:** Comedy **Time:** 110 min.

PostScript:
At the beginning of the film, Tenenbaum is evicted from the hotel where he's been living for decades. Broke, lonely and homeless, he seeks to rekindle his relationship with his estranged family. Unfortunately, he was so nasty that he needs a scheme to contact them again. He announces that he has stomach cancer and has only weeks left to live. . . and the ploy works! The power that the illness has on a family is nicely illustrated in the scene where he first tells his ex-wife that he's dying. She radiates sympathy and caring, and embraces him despite his many years of irresponsible behavior. Tenenbaum is immediately allowed to move back into the family home. He has a bedroom to himself, a personal attendant, and an impressive array of medical machines, ostensibly to ease his suffering and prolong his life. When confronted with a difficult issue, Royal slowly falls to the ground and puts a spoon between his teeth as if he is expecting to have a seizure. He asks for a barbiturate by name, giving an air of authenticity to his illness.

Dissociative Disorders

 # THE THREE FACES OF EVE

 Diagnosis Portrayed: Dissociative Identity Disorder
DSM-IV-TR Code: 300.14

 Accuracy Rating:
★★★/★★★

 Character's Name: Eve White/Eve Black/Jane
Actor's Name: Joanne Woodward

 Signs & Symptoms
Amnesia is too extensive to be considered ordinary forgetfulness
At least two of the alters recurrently take control of the person's behavior
Two or more distinct identities or personality states (alters) are present

 Year of Release: 1957 **Country:** USA
Language: English   **Genre:** Drama **Time:** 91 min.

PostScript:
Eve White is a dowdy, sullen woman who is referred to psychiatrist Dr. Luther (Lee J. Cobb). She had been experiencing splitting headaches, which preceded a "spell" lasting several hours, and for which Eve had no recollection. After the initial visit with Dr. Luther, Eve has a period of several months where these episodes do not recur. Then one day several dresses and pairs of shoes are delivered to her home, purportedly ordered by Eve. However, she can't recall purchasing these luxuries and her husband didn't buy them as surprise gifts. When Eve returns to see Dr. Luther, the prospect of having a mental illness is so upsetting for Eve that she dissociates and an alter emerges — Eve Black. This personality state is aware of everything that happens to Eve White, but does not have the ability to emerge on her own. Eve Black is allergic to her nylons, smokes cigarettes, likes to dance, and is rather flirtatious.

Reel to Real: **Psychiatric Conditions in Cinema**

NURSE BETTY

Diagnosis Portrayed: Dissociative Fugue
DSM-IV-TR Code: 300.13

Accuracy Rating:
★★★/★★★

Character's Name: Betty Sizemore
Actor's Name: Renée Zellweger

Signs & Symptoms
Assumes a new identity
Confusion about personal identity
Sudden, unplanned travel away from home or customary place of work
The unplanned travel is accompanied by an inability to recall one's past

Year of Release: 2000 **Country:** Germany/USA
Language: English **Genre:** Comedy **Time:** 100 min.

PostScript:

Betty is a waitress in a small town in Kansas. Her husband Del (Aaron Eckhart), finding that the used car business isn't profitable enough, unwittingly tries to sell stolen drugs back to the hoodlums from whom they were taken. Two assassins are sent to recover the goods, and in the process Del is murdered in his own home in front of Betty. Betty is a devotee of a soap opera, and is enamored of one of its stars, Dr. David Ravell (Greg Kinnear). Overwhelmed by the brutal slaying of her husband, Betty develops amnesia. She psychologically replaces the loss of her husband with the latest plot twist in the soap opera, which becomes her new reality. She is correctly diagnosed at the police station as being in a dissociative state. The day after Del's death she writes him a letter announcing their separation. Betty then heads off to Hollywood to help her beloved Dr. Ravell through his (fictional) crisis.

Sexual and Gender Identity Disorders

 ## WOODSMAN, THE

 Diagnosis Portrayed: Pedophilia
DSM-IV-TR Code: 302.2

 Accuracy Rating:
★★★/★★★

 Character's Name: Walter Rossworth
Actor's Name: Kevin Bacon

 Signs & Symptoms
Intense, recurrent sexually arousing fantasies involving children
Person is at least 16 years, and is 5 years older than the object of the fantasy

 Year of Release: 2004 **Country:** USA
Language: English **Genre:** Drama **Time:** 87 min.

PostScript:
Walter is a convicted pedophile who is attracted to pubescent females. This movie chronicles his life just after he is paroled. Having very few available places to live, he ironically ends up with a view of a grade school playground from his apartment window. Walter is offered a job because of his previous good work record and tries diligently to keep to himself and leave his conviction a secret. He accepts the advances of Vicki (Kyra Sedgwick) and they begin a relationship. She eventually is told about his past, but before she can react to the information, Walter asks her to leave because he feels that if she accepts what he has done, she must be sicker than he is. Walter eventually learns that Vicki was sexually abused by all three of her brothers, but despite this holds them in high esteem for the men that they have become. She sees the good in Walter, though he struggles with his fantasies when things become difficult at work or when the Sergeant Lucas (Mos Def), the detective monitoring his progress, visits to intimidate him.

Reel to Real: **Psychiatric Conditions in Cinema**

BLUE VELVET

Diagnosis Portrayed: Sexual Masochism/Sexual Sadism
DSM-IV-TR Code: 302.83/302.84

Accuracy Rating:
★★★/★★★

Character's Name: Dorothy Vallens/Frank Booth
Actor's Name: Isabella Rossellini/Dennis Hopper

Signs & Symptoms: Recurrent, intense, and arousing fantasies, urges or behaviors of being humiliated, beaten, bound, or otherwise made to suffer (masochism)
Enjoyment in inflicting physical violence, pain, humiliation, or harsh discipline on others, in which the suffering of the victim is erotically stimulating (sadism)

Year of Release: 1986 **Country:** USA
Language: English **Genre:** Crime **Time:** 120 min.

PostScript:
Jeffrey Beaumont (Kyle MacLachlan) becomes intrigued with the unusual events in his town and decides to become an amateur detective. His first step is to sneak into Dorothy's apartment. He makes a noise while hiding in the closet, and she arms herself with a knife and upon finding him, orders him to explain what he's doing. Thus begins a series of erotic events that portray a variety of paraphilias. In the first one, Dorothy orders Jeffrey to strip at knife point. Dorothy alternates between being dominant/sadistic and submissive/masochistic. Dorothy and Jeffrey are interrupted by the unexpected arrival of Frank Booth, who is an aggressive sadist who then dominates Dorothy.

Sexual and Gender Identity Disorders

JUST LIKE A WOMAN

Diagnosis Portrayed: Transvestic Fetishism
DSM-IV-TR Code: 302.3

Accuracy Rating:
★★★/★★★

Character's Name: Geraldine/Gerald Tilson
Actor's Name: Adrian Pasdar

Signs & Symptoms: Recurrent, sexually arousing fantasies, urges, or behaviors of a male to dress in women's attire

Year of Release: 1992 **Country:** UK
Language: English **Genre:** Comedy **Time:** 105 min.

PostScript:
Tilson is an American investment banker working in England. He is handsome, successful, and both a husband and father. His wife and children return early from a trip and he scrambles to get home before they do, but he arrives too late. Gerald's wife discovers women's clothing — particularly lingerie — in their home. She assumes that Gerald is having an affair and ends their marriage without hearing his explanation. Gerald has transvestic fetishism, and the clothes are his. He has dressed up as a woman all of his life, but hasn't told his wife and cannot bring himself to tell her even though it might save his marriage. Gerald moves into a boarding home run by Monica (Julie Walters). One evening Monica notices a woman visiting Gerald's apartment and asks him about her. He decides to trust Monica with his transvestic interests, and after a short period of adjustment, she accepts Gerald's practices and actually finds them stimulating. Gerald makes it clear that he is strictly heterosexual, and has no difficulty being intimate with Monica when he is able to dress according to his desires.

Reel to Real: **Psychiatric Conditions in Cinema**

SLIVER

Diagnosis Portrayed: Voyeurism
DSM-IV-TR Code: 302.82

Accuracy Rating:
★★★/★★★

Character's Name: Zeke Hawkins
Actor's Name: William Baldwin

Signs & Symptoms: Recurrent fantasy, urge, or behavior of watching an unsuspecting person disrobe or engage in sexual activity

Year of Release: 1993 **Country:** USA
Language: English **Genre:** Romance **Time:** 108 min.

PostScript:
Carly Norris (Sharon Stone) is a New York City book editor whose tenancy application is approved for an apartment in a "sliver" building so quickly that it surprises even her. What Carly doesn't realize at the time is that the building is owned by Hawkins, one of the other tenants. He is a voyeur's voyeur, and instead of hoping for a glimpse of people's private lives, he's hidden cameras and microphones in each apartment. He spends much of his time in a custom-built, multi-million dollar control room where he monitors and records other tenants' activities. Hawkins anonymously leaves a telescope in Carly's apartment, and is delighted when she scans other apartment buildings for interesting activities. Carly holds a cocktail party for her co-workers, one of whom delights in using the telescope to find a couple making love with the lights on. Many of the guests at the party wait their turn to watch the amorous couple. At the end of the evening, Carly has another look at the couple, and is surprised to find that they are sitting in the nude on their bed scanning other apartment buildings with their own telescope.

Sexual and Gender Identity Disorders

ADVENTURES OF PRISCILLA, QUEEN OF THE DESERT, THE

Diagnosis Portrayed: Gender Identity Disorder
DSM-IV-TR Code: 302.85

Accuracy Rating:
★★★ / ★★★

Character's Name: Bernadette
Actor's Name: Terence Stamp

Signs & Symptoms:
A strong and persistent cross-gender identification
Persistent discomfort with one's assigned sex

Year of Release: 1994 **Country:** Australia
Language: English **Genre:** Comedy **Time:** 104 min.

PostScript:
Priscilla is the name given to the bus used by three performers whose act consists of lip syncing and choreographing a variety of disco hits. The trio consists of Tick (Hugo Weaving), Adam (Guy Pearce), and Bernadette. Adam is a gay man, Tick is bisexual, and Bernadette is a transsexual. Bernadette, formerly named Ralph, is shown in a flashback switching Christmas presents with his sister so that he could play with the doll that was intended for her. He then became a she after having sexual reassignment surgery and takes hormones to develop breasts and some feminine sexual characteristics. Bernadette clearly defines herself as a woman and is always seen with a wig, make-up, and feminine clothing. She seeks to engage in heterosexual relationships with men. She expects to be treated like a lady, and accepts the flowers and kind attention of a rugged outback dweller named Bob (Bill Hunter).

Reel to Real: Psychiatric Conditions in Cinema

 # BEST LITTLE GIRL IN THE WORLD, THE

 Diagnosis Portrayed: Anorexia Nervosa
DSM-IV-TR Code: 307.1

 Accuracy Rating:
★★★/★★★

 Character's Name: Casey Powell
Actor's Name: Jennifer Jason Leigh

 Signs & Symptoms:
Amenorrhea
Denial of the serious medical consequences of being underweight
Distortion in body image such that the person perceives him or herself to be overweight
Intense fear of becoming fat despite being underweight
Refusal to maintain body weight at least at 85% of expected for age and height
Undue influence of body shape on self-evaluation

 Year of Release: 1981 **Country:** USA
Language: English **Genre:** Drama **Time:** 100 min.

PostScript:
Casey's ballet instructor praises her abilities but advises her to lose weight if she is serious about dancing. As Casey leaves the studio she is reminded not to drink any milk shakes. Casey buys a fashion magazine and begins to focus on the thinness of the models, and soon after starts to diet and exercise. Casey constantly evaluates her appearance in a full-length mirror that hangs behind her bedroom door. She has a bathroom to herself and begins to vomit there without being detected.

Eating Disorders

 ## A Secret Between Friends

 Diagnosis Portrayed: Bulimia Nervosa
DSM-IV-TR Code: 307.51

 Accuracy Rating:
★★★/★★★

 Character's Name: Lexi Archer/Jennifer Harnsberger
Actor's Name: Katie Wright/Marley Shelton

 Signs & Symptoms:
Binge eating behavior
Feeling a lack of control over one's eating during the binge
Recurrent, inappropriate compensatory behavior
Self-esteem and self-evaluation are strongly influenced by body shape and weight

 Year of Release: 1996 **Country:** USA/Canada
Language: English   **Genre:** Drama **Time:** 96 min.

PostScript:
This movie is also known as *When Friendship Kills*. Lexi is a new student at high school, having been forced to relocate by her parent's separation. She is a good athlete and makes the school volleyball team. Lexi develops a fast friendship with the team's star player, Jennifer. On one occasion when Lexi visits Jennifer, they "raid the fridge." The scene depicted afterwards is classic for binge eating. There are several empty containers of ice cream, cookies, candy, and potato chips that litter the table top — all of them empty. The two girls recline next to one another on a couch and are clearly uncomfortable because they've consumed too much food, and appear to have been unable to stop before they reached that point. Jennifer then introduces Lexi to purging.

Reel to Real: Psychiatric Conditions in Cinema

BULWORTH

Diagnosis Portrayed: Primary Insomnia
DSM-IV-TR Code: 307.42

Accuracy Rating:
★/★★★

Character's Name: Senator Jay Billington Bulworth
Actor's Name: Warren Beatty

Signs & Symptoms: Predominant difficulty is initiating sleep
Sleep disturbance causes significant impairment in important areas of functioning

Year of Release: 1998 **Country:** USA
Language: English **Genre:** Comedy **Time:** 108 min.

PostScript:
Bulworth is a California senator seeking re-election. Somewhere during the last week of his campaign he has an emotional meltdown, which occurs before the film begins. When we first see him, he hasn't slept for two nights and is feeling sluggish. Though he has several important decisions to make, Bulworth sits in his office staring blankly at a TV that among other things, plays his own commercials. Bulworth then flies cross-country, drinks alcohol and uses marijuana, all of which worsen his sleeping problem. Even without the influence of jet lag and substance abuse, Bulworth is a "sleep drunkard" and is disinhibited. He makes poor decisions, alienates many supporters, and ruins his reputation. These consequences are good examples of the social and occupational impairment that is specified in the DSM-IV-TR criteria. In this movie, it is difficult to ascribe all of Bulworth's erratic behavior to sleep deprivation. He does get a full night's sleep on the last day depicted in the film and appears to be back to his usual "right of center" self.

Sleep Disorders

 # My Own Private Idaho

 Diagnosis Portrayed: Narcolepsy
DSM-IV-TR Code: 347

 Accuracy Rating:
★★★/★★★

 Character's Name: Mike Waters
Actor's Name: River Phoenix

 Signs & Symptoms:
Irresistible sleep attacks of refreshing sleep
Recurrent intrusions of rapid eye muscle (REM) sleep into the transition between sleep and wakefulness
Sudden bilateral loss of muscle tone (cataplexy), often at times when intense emotions are being expressed

 Year of Release: 1991 **Country:** USA
Language: English **Genre:** Drama **Time:** 104 min.

PostScript:
The opening image in this movie is a classic portrayal of narcolepsy. Waters is a troubled young man who makes his living in the sex trade. When we first see him, he is stranded on a desolate Idaho highway. No vehicles approach for an extended period of time and he has a narcoleptic episode that leaves him asleep in the middle of the road. Waters has a sleep-onset REM episode, which is nicely depicted by his eyes moving back and forth as soon as he falls asleep. Waters does not receive treatment for his sleep attacks and continues to have them on a daily basis. In another scene, he becomes emotionally overwrought while preparing to have sexual relations with a woman, falls to the floor in her bedroom, and needs to be carried out by a friend.

Reel to Real: Psychiatric Conditions in Cinema

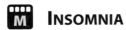

INSOMNIA

Diagnosis Portrayed: Circadian Rhythm Sleep Disorder
DSM-IV-TR Code: 307.45

Accuracy Rating:
★★/★★★

Character's Name: Will Dormer
Actor's Name: Al Pacino

Signs & Symptoms: Persistent pattern of sleep disruption that leads to insomnia and is due to a mismatch between environmental requirements and the person's circadian sleep-wake schedule
Social, occupational, or other areas of function are significantly impaired by the sleep disturbance

Year of Release: 2002 **Country:** USA/Canada
Language: English **Genre:** Thriller **Time:** 118 min.

PostScript:
This film was originally a 1997 Norwegian release and was redone in 2002, which is the version presented here. Dormer is a Los Angeles detective who flies to Alaska to help solve a murder. In northern regions there is sunlight for most of the day during the summer and Dormer has considerable difficulty making this adjustment. He cannot sleep because of the persistent light streaming into his hotel room. Dormer goes for almost six days without sleep and becomes progressively more disorganized and makes a number of errors in his investigation. This portrayal is less than entirely accurate because there are many things plaguing Dormer's conscience that would impair his sleep, not just the increased number of hours of daylight.

Sleep Disorders

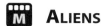

Aliens

Diagnosis Portrayed: Nightmare Disorder
DSM-IV-TR Code: 307.47

Accuracy Rating:
★★★/★★★

Character's Name: Ellen Ripley
Actor's Name: Sigourney Weaver

Signs & Symptoms:
Dream experience causes significant distress or impairment in functioning
Repeated awakenings from the major sleep period with detailed recall of the frightening dream
Upon awakening, the person is quickly able to orient himself or herself and is alert

Year of Release: 1986 **Country:** USA/UK
Language: English **Genre:** Sci-Fi **Time:** 137 min.

PostScript:
Aliens is the first sequel to the 1979 release of Alien. Ellen and her cat Jonesy are the only survivors of an attack by a alien creature. Ellen barely manages to get into an escape pod, and then is in "hypersleep" for over 50 years before she is found. Upon awakening, she is interviewed extensively about her experiences and the loss of her space ship. She begins to have distressing dreams of her harrowing experiences and close brush with death. She clearly remembers what her dream experiences involve, and recognizes immediately upon awakening what has occurred. Ellen is distraught and distracted by her nightmares and ends up working at a level far below her abilities. . . until she agrees to go back to the planet where the alien was discovered.

Reel to Real: **Psychiatric Conditions in Cinema**

DONNIE DARKO

Diagnosis Portrayed: Sleepwalking Disorder
DSM-IV-TR Code: 307.46

Accuracy Rating:
★★★/★★★

Character's Name: Donnie Darko
Actor's Name: Jake Gyllenhaal

Signs & Symptoms:
Amnesia for the episode of sleepwalking
Full recovery of mental functions upon awakening from the sleepwalking episode
Repeated episodes of rising from bed during sleep and walking about
Unresponsive to the environment while sleepwalking

Year of Release: 2001 **Country:** USA
Language: English **Genre:** Drama **Time:** 113 min.

PostScript:
Prior to the film beginning, Darko has started some type of psychiatric medication and has regular therapy sessions. At precisely midnight he sits up in bed, slowly gets dressed, and leaves the house. He walks down the street and eventually falls asleep on a putting green at a nearby golf course. Sleepwalking usually occurs in the first third of sleep, so his episode at midnight is consistent with this disorder. He also has no idea the next morning how he got to the golf course. Some people remember fragments of what they were experiencing while sleepwalking but it is more typical to not remember anything. The activities that people engage in while sleepwalking are fairly routine.

Impulse-Control Disorders

 # PUNCH-DRUNK LOVE

 Diagnosis Portrayed: Intermittent Explosive Disorder
DSM-IV-TR Code: 312.34

 Accuracy Rating:
★★★/★★★

 Character's Name: Barry Egan
Actor's Name: Adam Sandler

 Signs & Symptoms: Episodes of aggressive action that result in serious destruction of property
Episodes of aggression are far out of proportion to the factors that precipitate them

 Year of Release: 2002 **Country:** USA
Language: English **Genre:** Comedy **Time:** 95 min.

PostScript:
Egan owns a business selling novelty plungers. While repeatedly trying to close a deal, he receives phone calls from each of his seven sisters who implore him to attend a birthday party. At the party, Barry is gently ribbed about some of his boyhood antics. Ironically, it is the teasing about previous angry outbursts that cause him to again lose control of his temper, and Barry kicks out the glass from a sliding door. Later in the film, Barry meets Lena (Emily Watson), a friend of one of his sisters, and has dinner with her. In the course of their conversation, Lena mentions something she heard about one of Barry's childhood outbursts. He calmly excuses himself and then proceeds to trash the men's washroom. After doing so, he sits down and resumes their polite dinner conversation. Barry does not have an irritable disposition, nor a personality disorder, and doesn't seem to be suffering from another condition that would account for his destructive outbursts.

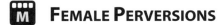

FEMALE PERVERSIONS

Diagnosis Portrayed: Kleptomania
DSM-IV-TR Code: 312.32

Accuracy Rating:
★★★/★★★

Character's Name: Maddie Stephens
Actor's Name: Amy Madigan

Signs & Symptoms:
Irresistible impulses to steal items that are not needed for personal use or for their value
Tension mounts before the theft and reduces immediately afterwards

Year of Release: 1996 **Country:** Germany/USA
Language: English **Genre:** Drama **Time:** 119 min.

PostScript:
While this film does have an erotic focus, the title of this movie stems from the "perversity" of having to curtail the expression of one's sexuality to the confines of what is considered socially acceptable, rather than for any specific act being portrayed. The kleptomaniac in this film is Maddie, a graduate student who is just days from defending her thesis. She comes from at least an upper-middle class background and has a sister who is a highly successful lawyer. Maddie enters a lingerie store and steals a scarf by slowly wrapping it around her neck. Spurred by the excitement of the successful theft of the scarf, she then asks the clerk to look for an item in another color and impulsively steals a garter belt by concealing it in her pants. Maddie then leaves the store, and while staring right back at the entrance, removes the garter and throws it in a garbage can. We later learn that she has taken many items that are not useful to her, such as a dozen hammers and children's clothes.

Impulse-Control Disorders

 # Owning Mahowny

 Diagnosis Portrayed: Pathological Gambling
DSM-IV-TR Code: 312.31

 Accuracy Rating:
★★★/★★★

 Character's Name: Dan Mahowny
Actor's Name: Philip Seymour Hoffman

 Signs & Symptoms:
Chases gambling losses
Committed illegal acts to obtain money
Gambles with increasing amounts of money to achieve the desired effect
Irritable when attempting to stop
Jeopardizes relationships and employment because of gambling
Lies about extent of gambling
Preoccupied with gambling

 Year of Release: 2003 **Country:** Canada/UK
Language: English **Genre:** Crime **Time:** 104 min.

PostScript:
Mahowny is a rising star in a large bank and gets a promotion that gives him access to funds without needing his supervisor's approval. Mahowny is addicted to gambling before the movie begins, but this development gives him the chance to bet (and lose) much larger sums of money. He is the antithesis of the flashy gambler. Mahowny eschews attention, alcohol, and the female escort provided by the casino for high rollers. His demeanor so rarely changes that the video surveillance operators at the casino call him "Ice Man." All of this belies a man who is in desperately in denial about his problem, defrauding his employer of millions of dollars, and jeopardizing his relationship and his future.

Reel to Real: **Psychiatric Conditions in Cinema**

BACKDRAFT

Diagnosis Portrayed: Pyromania
DSM-IV-TR Code: 312.33

Accuracy Rating:
★★★/★★★

Character's Name: Ronald Bartel
Actor's Name: Donald Sutherland

Signs & Symptoms:
Affective arousal before setting the fire
Deliberate fire setting on more than one occasion and not for financial gain
Fascination with fire and its consequences

Year of Release: 1991 **Country:** USA
Language: English **Genre:** Action **Time:** 132 min.

PostScript:
Bartel is an imprisoned pyromaniac in this film. Although he did engage in committing arson, he was clearly enamored of fire before hiring out his talents. Bartel keeps track of major fires with the avidity that collectors have for trading cards of their favorite athletes. Bartel instantly recognizes the name of Brian McCaffrey (Stephen Baldwin) from a magazine cover showing McCaffrey as a child at the scene of a fire holding the helmet of his father (who perished in the blaze). Bartel refers to fire as "the animal" and has pathological reverence for it. Bartel is so fixated on fire and its consequences that he admits at his parole hearing that he likes to burn people, and if given the chance, he would burn the whole world. Fire investigator Donald Rimgale (Robert De Niro) tells McCaffrey that fire is alive — it breathes, and eats, and hates. Furthering Rimgale's anthropomorphization of fire, Bartel asks McCaffrey if the fire "looked" at him and was entranced to hear that it did.

Impulse-Control Disorders

 ## Dirty Filthy Love

 Diagnosis Portrayed: Trichotillomania
DSM-IV-TR Code: 312.39

 Accuracy Rating:
★★★/★★★

 Character's Name: Charlotte
Actor's Name: Shirley Henderson

 Signs & Symptoms: Increasing tension before pulling hair and gratification afterwards
Recurrent pulling out of one's hair leading to noticeable hair loss

 Year of Release: 2004 **Country:** UK
Language: English **Genre:** Drama **Time:** 120 min.

PostScript:
This is a made-for-TV movie that is widely available commercially. The main character in this film is Mark Furness (Michael Sheen), an architect whose life takes a turn for the worse when his wife leaves him. Furness suffers from Tourette's disorder and obsessive-compulsive disorder, both of which worsen and become disabling for him, particularly in social contexts (such as when he tries to get his job back after an extended leave of absence). In order to seek help, Furness discovers a self-help group run by Charlotte for people with OCD. She is far more functional in this movie that he is, running a health food store/organic bakery, and does a great job with the group. Charlotte's hair seems to be forever in her face, often obscuring it from the viewer. She chews on her hair in a couple of scenes, particularly when she gets a bit stressed by her romantic interest in Furness. Close to the end of the film, she helps Furness confront his estranged wife, and in the process, Charlotte's wig gets pulled off revealing the extent of her trichotillomania.

Reel to Real: Psychiatric Conditions in Cinema

 # CAINE MUTINY, THE

 Diagnosis Portrayed: Paranoid Personality Disorder
DSM-IV-TR Code: 301.1

 Accuracy Rating:
★★★/★★★

 Character's Name: Lt. Cmdr. Philip Francis Queeg
Actor's Name: Humphrey Bogart

 Signs & Symptoms:
Perceives attacks on his character when there are none intended
Preoccupied with the loyalty of his crew
Reads hidden meanings into things
Reluctant to confide in, or trust, others
Suspects, without justification, that others are deceiving him

 Year of Release: 1954 **Country:** USA
Language: English **Genre:** Drama **Time:** 124 min.

PostScript:
The U.S.S. Caine, a fictitious W.W. II minesweeper, is described by her initial skipper Lt. Cmdr. DeVriess (Tom Tully) as a "beaten up tub" in the "junkyard navy." The ship and crew are noticeably in need of an overhaul when Queeg takes command. Queeg is focused on order and obedience and views every small transgression as a deliberate challenge to his authority. Shortly after taking command, he berates a sailor for leaving his shirttail out and, while so engaged, steams over a tow line. He cannot accept that he has done something wrong and files a report insisting that the equipment was faulty. Many incidents follow where Queeg's paranoid rants loses him the affection and respect of the officers and crew, particularly after strip search is ordered as part of an investigation to discover the fate of a missing quart of strawberries.

Personality Disorders

 ## MAN WHO WASN'T THERE, THE

 Diagnosis Portrayed: Schizoid Personality Disorder
DSM-IV-TR Code: 301.20

 Accuracy Rating:
★★★/★★★

Character's Name: Ed Crane
Actor's Name: Billy Bob Thornton

 Signs & Symptoms:
Emotionally cold and detached
Few interests or activities
Indifferent to the input of other people
Lack of interest in sexual activities

 Year of Release: 2001 **Country:** UK/USA
Language: English **Genre:** Crime **Time:** 116 min.

PostScript:
Crane is a barber who is very content with his place in life being "second chair" to the owner. He is married to Doris (Frances McDormand), with whom he shares a rather lackluster relationship. Crane is dry, laconic, and emotionally flat. He says little to anyone, including his wife, and she drifts into having an affair with Big Dave Brewster (James Gandolfini). Crane commits manslaughter, learns that his wife is pregnant, and has several other significant events happen to him, yet he cannot muster the fortitude to stand up for himself or the energy to try to correct things, hence the name of the movie. He is eventually executed for a crime he didn't commit, and he faces this event with his customary equanimity and indifference. Although his trial was at once going strongly in his favor, Crane gets a new lawyer and for no apparent reason, ends up pleading guilty. As his plea was being discussed, Crane just watches it happen and passively agrees with everyone else, making his presence known in as few words as possible.

Reel to Real: **Psychiatric Conditions in Cinema**

 # MAN WHO WASN'T THERE, THE

 Diagnosis Portrayed: Schizotypal Personality Disorder
DSM-IV-TR Code: 301.22

 Accuracy Rating:
★★★/★★★

 Character's Name: Ann Nirdlinger Brewster
Actor's Name: Katherine Borowitz

 Signs & Symptoms:
Affect is constricted and inappropriate
Behavior is eccentric and peculiar
Odd beliefs that influence her behavior and are inconsistent with cultural norms
Odd thinking and speech
Social anxiety that does not diminish with familiarity
Suspicious and paranoid ideas
Unusual perceptual experiences

 Year of Release: 2001   **Country:** UK/USA
Language: English   **Genre:** Crime   **Time:** 116 min.

PostScript:
Ann is the heiress of a large department store, but has left the operations of it to her husband, Big Dave. There are two scenes in this movie that beautifully demonstrate schizotypal traits. The first occurs when Ann and Dave visit Ed and Doris Crane. Ann is oblivious to the rampant flirtation going between her husband and Doris. The second occurs when she discusses Big Dave's death with Ed. She isn't there to seek solace or even any sort of explanation, but to tell Ed that Big Dave was never the same after an alien abduction had occurred several summers previously, and that she blames this for Big Dave's untimely death.

Personality Disorders

 ## Man Bites Dog

 Diagnosis Portrayed: Antisocial Personality Disorder
DSM-IV-TR Code: 301.7

 Accuracy Rating:

★★★/★★★

 Character's Name: Ben
Actor's Name: Benoît Poelvoorde

 Signs & Symptoms:
Aggressiveness and irritability
Consistent irresponsibility
Deceitful acts, such as lying and conning others
Lack of remorse for criminal acts
Reckless disregard for the welfare and safety of others
Repeated acts that are illegal and grounds for arrest

 Year of Release: 1993 **Country:** Belgium
Language: French **Genre:** Comedy **Time:** 95 min.

PostScript:
This movie is shot in a black-and-white "mockumentary" format. Ben is an antisocial's antisocial, a machine driven by predatory instincts and guiltless exploitation of those around him. He is a social parasite, making his living by preying on elderly pensioners, postal employees, and anyone availing him the slightest opportunity. Interspersed with his acts of extreme violence, Ben speaks eloquently into the camera about love, life, philosophy, etc. He expresses admiration and sympathy for a man that he has just killed, saying that he was too young to be forced into employment. In another memorable scene, Ben describes scientific strategies for disposing of a variety of body types in a river.

Reel to Real: Psychiatric Conditions in Cinema

 # SINGLE WHITE FEMALE

 Diagnosis Portrayed: Borderline Personality Disorder
DSM-IV-TR Code: 301.83

 Accuracy Rating:
★★★/★★★

 Character's Name: Hedra "Hedy" Carlson
Actor's Name: Jennifer Jason Leigh

 Signs & Symptoms:
Affective instability
Chronic feelings of emptiness
Difficulty controlling anger
Frantic efforts to avoid abandonment
Identity disturbance
Unstable, intense relationships

 Year of Release: 1992 **Country:** USA
Language: English **Genre:** Thriller **Time:** 107 min.

PostScript:
Allison (Bridget Fonda), hoping to find the perfect roommate, allows Hedra to move in with her. At first Hedra appears to fit the bill but what isn't revealed until later is that she is desperately searching for an unrealistic level of attachment to another person. Hedra leads a transient, chaotic existence. This movie provides an excellent example of identity disturbance and chronic feelings of emptiness. Hedra has no concept of being an individual; she idealizes Allison and defines herself as Allison's twin. If it were possible, she would merge with Allison. Hedra wears Allison's clothes, copies her hairstyle, and tries to keep her all to herself by interfering in Allison's relationship with boyfriend Sam (Steven Weber). The everyday things that she and Allison do together are of monumental importance to her, but she hides this under a self-effacing and bashful veneer. . . until Allison wants Sam to move in with her.

Personality Disorders

A STREETCAR NAMED DESIRE

Diagnosis Portrayed: Histrionic Personality Disorder
DSM-IV-TR Code: 301.50

Accuracy Rating:
★★★/★★★

Character's Name: Blanche DuBois
Actor's Name: Vivien Leigh

Signs & Symptoms:
Appearance is used to draw attention to self
Dramatic and theatrical expression of emotion
Easily suggestible
Interactions are inappropriately seductive or provocative
Speech is impressionistic and lacks detail

Year of Release: 1951 **Country:** USA
Language: English **Genre:** Drama **Time:** 122 min.

PostScript:
This movie is an adaptation of Tennessee Williams' play. Blanche flees the ruin she has brought to her life by moving in with her sister Stella (Kim Hunter) and brother-in-law Stanley (Marlon Brando). Blanche manages to become the center of attention and employs a repertoire of ways to accomplish this: animated gestures, a fast rate of speech, an air of superiority, fishing for compliments, distraction, and flirtatiousness. It is easy to see how Blanche interacts with others in maladaptive ways, and how the concept of a "disorder" applies to her personality characteristics. She's a charming wastrel who has squandered the family fortune, something she attempts to disguise by dumping piles of paper in front of Stanley when he presses her to account for what has happened.

Reel to Real: **Psychiatric Conditions in Cinema**

 # WALL STREET

 Diagnosis Portrayed: Narcissistic Personality Disorder
DSM-IV-TR Code: 301.81

 Accuracy Rating:
★★★/★★★

 Character's Name: Gordon Gekko
Actor's Name: Michael Douglas

 Signs & Symptoms:
Associates only with special or important people
Dramatic and theatrical expression of emotion
Excessive admiration is required
Exploitative
Grandiose sense of self importance
Preoccupied with unlimited success

 Year of Release: 1987 **Country:** USA
Language: English **Genre:** Crime **Time:** 125 min.

PostScript:
Gekko is a corporate raider who is adept at finding companies that he can liquidate for profit. He thrives on insider trading and manipulates Bud Fox (Charlie Sheen), a young stock broker, into believing that he (Bud) must engage in illegal activities in order to be special or important enough to take up Gekko's time. Gekko displays many of the cardinal features of NPD, particularly: exploitation of others; a sense of entitlement; a lack of empathy for the lives he ruins; and a preoccupation with unlimited success. This is well demonstrated during his "Greed is Good" speech to the board of directors of a company that he is planning to take over. Ultimately, Gekko's narcissism cannot bear the insult of Bud spurning him, and he spews out a confession that is taped by the police.

Personality Disorders

ZELIG

Diagnosis Portrayed: Avoidant Personality Disorder
DSM-IV-TR Code: 301.82

Accuracy Rating:
★★★/★★★

Character's Name: Leonard Zelig
Actor's Name: Woody Allen

Signs & Symptoms:
Preoccupied with being rejected
Sees self as inept and inferior
Shows restraint in relationships because of fear of shame or ridicule
Strong feelings of inadequacy
Unwilling to get involved with others unless acceptance is guaranteed

Year of Release: 1983 **Country:** USA
Language: English **Genre:** Comedy **Time:** 79 min.

PostScript:
Zelig is a human chameleon. He changes his appearance, accent, demeanor, and opinions to seamlessly blend in with the people around him. At a speak-easy party, he "morphs" from a white gangster into a black trumpet player in a matter of minutes. On another occasion he swells up to 250 lbs. in the presence of two portly gentlemen. Two French visitors induce him to grow a pencil-thin moustache and speak their language in a passable manner. Zelig is eventually brought to medical attention and becomes the principal focus of the psychiatrist Eudora Fletcher (Mia Farrow). In her company, Zelig assumes the appearance, bearing, and vocabulary of a colleague and identifies himself as a doctor. Under hypnosis, he explains to her that he changes himself around others because he wants to be safe and to be liked.

Reel to Real: Psychiatric Conditions in Cinema

 ## DELICATE ART OF PARKING, THE

 Diagnosis Portrayed: Dependent Personality Disorder
DSM-IV-TR Code: 301.6

 Accuracy Rating:
★★★/★★★

 Character's Name: Grant Parker
Actor's Name: Fred Ewanuick

 Signs & Symptoms:
Difficulty disagreeing with others
Difficulty initiating projects on own due to a lack of self-confidence
Difficulty making decisions without excessive advice and reassurance
Goes to excessive lengths to obtain support or acceptance from others

 Year of Release: 2003 **Country:** Canada
Language: English **Genre:** Comedy **Time:** 86 min.

PostScript:
Parker is a parking enforcement officer in a large city and very proud of his job. He is the consummate "true believer" and parrots back the scripts from his training videos as if they are his own ideas for why he chose this line of work. Parker believes that people have a right to vent at him and accepts both verbal and physical abuse because he feels that it is an integral part of his job. He has a very strong attachment to his supervisor and mentor, Murray (Gary Jones). Murray was the leading ticketer and union steward before he mysteriously got injured, and Parker is more proud of being #2 compared to Murray than he would be to take over his spot. Parker needs a considerable amount of coaxing to even consider taking over Murray's union job, although he appears to be well qualified.

Personality Disorders

 # REMAINS OF THE DAY, THE

 Diagnosis Portrayed: Obsessive-Compulsive Pers. Dis.
DSM-IV-TR Code: 301.4

 Accuracy Rating:
★★★/★★★

 Character's Name: James Stevens
Actor's Name: Anthony Hopkins

 Signs & Symptoms:
Preoccupied with details, rules, and order
Excessively devoted to work and productivity to the exclusion of leisure activities and friendships
Reluctant to delegate tasks
Rigid and stubborn

 Year of Release: 1993 **Country:** UK/USA
Language: English **Genre:** Drama **Time:** 134 min.

PostScript:
Stevens is the prototypical English butler: prim, meticulous, and utterly controlled. He is perpetually at work, saying that he can only feel content when he has done all he can to be of service to his employer. Stevens reads not for enjoyment, but to further his command of the English language. Miss Kenton (Emma Thompson) is hired as a housekeeper at the beginning of the film and develops an affection for Stevens that he also feels but cannot bring himself to disclose. Many of his rigid traits are highlighted against her humanistic and compassionate ways. In one scene, Stevens' father, who is employed as the under-butler, is dying and the younger Stevens refuses to leave his post. When Stevens finally takes a break, his father has passed away. Unable to demonstrate any emotion upon seeing his father's body, Stevens chooses instead to attend to a visiting dignitary's blisters.

Reel to Real: Psychiatric Conditions in Cinema

I Am Sam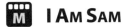

Diagnosis Portrayed: Mild Mental Retardation
DSM-IV-TR Code: 317

Accuracy Rating:
★★★/★★★

Character's Name: Sam Dawson
Actor's Name: Sean Penn

Signs & Symptoms: Impairments in:
- Communication
- Functional academic skills
- Home living
- Self care
- Social/interpersonal skills

Significantly subaverage mental functioning

Year of Release: 2001 **Country:** USA
Language: English **Genre:** Drama **Time:** 132 min.

PostScript:
Dawson is a man with mild mental retardation who functions at about the level of a seven-year old. At the beginning of the film, he is gainfully employed, lives independently, and manages his life in a functional manner until he becomes a single parent. The stresses and strains of raising a child highlight Sam's limitations in this new role, and he is eventually brought to the attention of children's protective services and the courts. In the audio commentary on the DVD, the director indicates how much research went into this film. Parts of the story were pieced together from actual experiences of people with psychiatric disorders. Two of Sam's close friends, Brad (Brad Silverman) and Joe (Joseph Rosenberg) are actors with actual disabilities.

Child & Adolescent Psychiatric Disorders

What's Eating Gilbert Grape

Diagnosis Portrayed: Moderate Mental Retardation
DSM-IV-TR Code: 318.0

Accuracy Rating:
★★★/★★★

Character's Name: Arnie Grape
Actor's Name: Leonardo DiCaprio

Signs & Symptoms:
Impairments in:
- Communication
- Functional academic skills
- Home living
- Leisure
- Safety
- Self care
- Self direction
- Social/interpersonal skills
- Work

Significantly subaverage mental functioning

Year of Release: 1993 **Country:** USA
Language: English **Genre:** Drama **Time:** 118 min.

PostScript:
Arnie suffered from a serious illness when he was born and as a result was not expected to live past the age of ten. At the beginning of the film he is just days shy of his 18th birthday. Arnie has managed to develop physically but suffers from moderate mental retardation. Arnie is a handful and requires constant attention from his siblings to keep him out of serious trouble. Left unsupervised, Arnie likes to climb things, his favorite structure being the town water tower.

Reel to Real: Psychiatric Conditions in Cinema

SECRET, THE

Diagnosis Portrayed: Reading Disorder
DSM-IV-TR Code: 315.00

Accuracy Rating:
★★★/★★★

Character's Name: Mike Dunmore/Danny Dunmore
Actor's Name: Kirk Douglas/Jesse R. Tendler

Signs & Symptoms: Academic, social and occupational roles are interfered with because of the difficulty with reading
Reading achievement is substantially below the level expected

Year of Release: 1992 **Country:** USA
Language: English **Genre:** Drama **Time:** 120 min.

PostScript:
Mike is a recent widower. He is a well-respected member of his community and a loving grandfather to Danny. Mike does a few unusual things: he needs to be told how to find a sewing kit by color alone, he gives Danny a "get well'" card for his birthday, and asks for a long string of items that are not on the menu at a restaurant. Danny ad-libs his way through a parents' day event at school, trades artwork for an essay, and gets caught cheating on an exam. Distracted widower? A kid learning to cut corners at an early age? Or is there a connection between these events? The answer is the family secret — both Mike and Danny suffer from dyslexia, which prevents them from being able to read and write properly. Mike was able to get by when his wife took care of all his written needs, so it is her absence from this role that brings to life his deficits. Mike is a master at being able to cover for his dyslexia, until he gets pressure to run for a seat on the town council.

Child & Adolescent Psychiatric Disorders

NELL

Diagnosis Portrayed: Phonological Disorder
DSM-IV-TR Code: 315.39

Accuracy Rating:
★★/★★★

Character's Name: Nell Kellty
Actor's Name: Jodie Foster

Signs & Symptoms:
Failure to use developmentally appropriate speech sounds for age and dialect
Social communication is significantly affected

Year of Release: 1994 **Country:** USA
Language: English **Genre:** Drama **Time:** 113 min.

PostScript:
In an isolated part of North Carolina it was thought that a woman lived alone for many years. After her death, it was discovered that she had twin daughters, one of whom (Nell) was still alive. Nell's mother suffered a stroke years earlier and, having subsequently become aphasic, had marked difficulty with articulation. Nell speaks in a seemingly unintelligible manner using utterances that are a combination of a private language that she spoke with her sister and imitation of her mother's aphasic speech. The technical term for this condition is *idioglossia*, which is also the name of the play on which this movie is based. This condition has also been called *cryptophasia*, *twin talk* and *twin speech*. While this is an outstanding movie, it is not that accurate a portrayal because of the circumstances under which Nell learned to speak — given that she does learn to speak English fluently, she clearly does have intact comprehension and speech abilities.

Reel to Real: Psychiatric Conditions in Cinema

[M] A FISH CALLED WANDA

Diagnosis Portrayed: Stuttering
DSM-IV-TR Code: 307.0

Accuracy Rating:
★★/★★★

Character's Name: Ken Pile
Actor's Name: Michael Palin

Signs & Symptoms:
Broken words
Monosyllabic whole-word repetition
Sound prolongation
Syllable repetition
Words produced with physical tension

Year of Release: 1988 **Country:** USA/UK
Language: English **Genre:** Comedy **Time:** 108 min.

PostScript:
Pile is awkward, nervous and reclusive. Despite having a pronounced stammer and low self-esteem, he is one of the principals who plan a jewel heist. In the course of events, one of his co-conspirators (Wanda played by Jamie Lee Curtis) accepts his speech impediment, another (Otto played by Kevin Kline) ridicules him, and a third (Archie Leach played by John Cleese) is indifferent to it. The film received a wide range of attention from various stuttering advocacy groups. Michael Palin made donations to various agencies and went on to found a center for stammering children that bears his name.

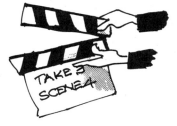

Child & Adolescent Psychiatric Disorders

Rain Man

Diagnosis Portrayed: Autistic Disorder
DSM-IV-TR Code: 299.00

Accuracy Rating:
★★★/★★★

Character's Name: Raymond Babbitt
Actor's Name: Dustin Hoffman

Signs & Symptoms:
Behavioral abnormalities:
- Inflexible adherence to routines
- Repetitive motor mannerisms
- Restricted patterns of interest

Communication deficits:
- Impaired conversation skills
- Stereotyped and repetitive language

Social skills deficits:
- Lack of social reciprocity
- Lack of spontaneous sharing of joy
- Failure to develop peer relationships

Year of Release: 1988   **Country:** USA
Language: English   **Genre:** Drama   **Time:** 133 min.

PostScript:
Charlie (Tom Cruise) seeks out his estranged brother Raymond after their father dies in order to acquire his sibling's share of the inheritance. Raymond has been institutionalized for years and displays many of the cardinal symptoms of autism. The behavioral, communication, and social interaction aspects are very well portrayed in this film. The single biggest potential inaccuracy is that Raymond's savant skills (primarily his incredible counting ability) are indeed rare and not something that is present in every person suffering from autistic disorder.

Reel to Real: Psychiatric Conditions in Cinema

 # MOZART AND THE WHALE

 Diagnosis Portrayed: Asperger's Disorder
DSM-IV-TR Code: 299.80

 Accuracy Rating:
★★★/★★★

 Character's Name: Josh Hartnett/Radha Mitchell
Actor's Name: Donald Morton/Isabelle Sorenson

 Signs & Symptoms:
Impairment in non-verbal behavior
Lack of social reciprocity
Motor mannerisms
Peer interactions are impaired
Restricted patterns of interest
Routines or rituals that are inflexible

 Year of Release: 2005 **Country:** USA
Language: English **Genre:** Romance **Time:** 92 min.

PostScript:
This movie is based on the true life experiences of two people that suffer from Asperger's disorder, albeit in significantly different ways. The title stems from the costumes they wore on their first date, which was on Hallowe'en. The movie is not to be confused with the similarly titled *The Squid and the Whale*, which has nothing to do with pervasive developmental disorders. Morton has Asperger's disorder, which has given him an incredible talent for numbers. In one scene he watches the time count down on a microwave oven and tells engaging stories about the numbers as they appear. He is relatively high functioning and actually runs a support group for people with various diagnoses. In this capacity he meets Isabelle, who is more of a free spirit and comfortable with setting the pace of the relationship. In this movie, she has fewer of the typical features of Asperger's than does Morton.

Child & Adolescent Psychiatric Disorders

 ## THUMBSUCKER

 Diagnosis Portrayed: Attention-Deficit Hyperactivity Disorder
DSM-IV-TR Code: 314.00

 Accuracy Rating:
★★/★★★

 Character's Name: Justin Cobb
Actor's Name: Lou Taylor Pucci

 Signs & Symptoms:
Avoids tasks requiring sustained attention
Blurts out answers in class
Difficulty organizing tasks
Fails to finish tasks
Talks excessively

 Year of Release: 2005 **Country:** USA
Language: English **Genre:** Comedy **Time:** 96 min.

PostScript:
At the beginning of this film, Cobb arguably suffers from the attention deficit aspect of this disorder. He daydreams constantly, isolates himself, and generally mismanages things to the point where he is miserable and can't seem to do much about it. He engages in a form of hypnosis performed by his über-hip dentist (zentistry?), Dr. Lyman (Keanu Reeves). When this doesn't work, he is diagnosed with ADHD by someone at his school and placed on methylphenidate (Ritalin®). Paradoxically, it is at this point that Cobb starts to display behaviors consistent with the hyperactivity aspect of this condition. In particular, he blurts out answers in class, acts as if he is driven by a motor/always on the go, and interrupts or intrudes on others. He performs much better at his school tasks, becomes the debating team champion, and manages to manipulate his way into a university acceptance.

Reel to Real: Psychiatric Conditions in Cinema

GOOD SON, THE

Diagnosis Portrayed: Conduct Disorder, Childhood-Onset Type
DSM-IV-TR Code: 312.81

Accuracy Rating:
★★★/★★★

Character's Name: Henry Evans
Actor's Name: Macaulay Culkin

Signs & Symptoms:
Aggression towards people and animals
Cruelty to people and animals
Deceitfulness
Threatens and intimidates others

Year of Release: 1993 **Country:** USA
Language: English **Genre:** Drama **Time:** 87 min.

PostScript:
Only Henry's age would preclude him from being diagnosed with antisocial personality disorder or severe psychopathy. The prototypic devil dressed up to appear like an angel, he undertakes many terrible activities in this movie, including murder. Henry kills a neighbor's dog with a crossbow, causes a serious pile-up on a highway with a dummy meant to look like a person, and intimidates or manipulates everyone around him. When his cousin Mark (Elijah Wood) comes to visit, Henry's sociopathic activities threaten to get exposed, but since Mark just suffered the loss of his mother, everyone just assumes he is responding to this loss with an active imagination. Henry goes on to try to poison his family and to kill his younger sister Connie (Quinn Culkin). The end of the film shows the extent of the depravity and cunning of this junior psychopath. Nothing he says can be taken at face value and he is a skilled liar and a very dangerous young person.

Child & Adolescent Psychiatric Disorders

YOUNG POISONER'S HANDBOOK, THE

Diagnosis Portrayed: Conduct Disorder, Adolescent-Onset Type
DSM-IV-TR Code: 312.82

Accuracy Rating:
★★★/★★★

Character's Name: Graham Young
Actor's Name: Hugh O'Connor

Signs & Symptoms:	Aggression towards people (poisoning) Deceitfulness Rights of others are ignored Serious violations of rules

Year of Release: 1995 **Country:** UK/Germany/France
Language: English **Genre:** Comedy **Time:** 99 min.

PostScript:
This movie is based on a true story of the "Teacup Poisoner" who was a British serial killer. This film depicts Young as having a flair for the macabre at an early age, which might have qualified him for the diagnosis of conduct disorder, childhood-onset type if more information was available. Young's principal activity of poisoning others gets into full swing when he is a teenager and had acquired the knowledge and means to poison others. He poisons a schoolmate in order to capitalize on the ensuing illness and steal the boy's girlfriend. Young is arrested at age 14 and charged with the poisoning death of his stepmother and attempted murder of his father. A prison sentence only serves to heighten Young's sociopathic tendencies, and when he is released he obtains work in a camera factory in order to get access to an ingredient in the shutter system — thallium, his poisoning agent of choice. He puts it in his co-workers' mugs, hence his moniker.

Reel to Real: **Psychiatric Conditions in Cinema**

UNDERTOW

Diagnosis Portrayed: Pica
DSM-IV-TR Code: 307.52

Accuracy Rating:
★★★/★★★

Character's Name: Tim Munn
Actor's Name: Devon Alan

Signs & Symptoms:
Age-inappropriate eating of non-nutritive substances
Non-nutritive substances are not culturally sanctioned to eat
Persistent eating of non-nutritive substances

Year of Release: 2004 **Country:** USA
Language: English **Genre:** Drama **Time:** 108 min.

Post Script:
Tim lives with his older brother Chris (Jamie Bell) and father John (Dermot Mulroney) on an isolated hog farm in Georgia. Tim and Chris' mother passes away before the film begins, and John decides to live a life of quiet seclusion as a result. Tim is thin for his age and shows his disinterest or difficulty in eating food at various points in the movie. He has been diagnosed with an "anxiety disorder," but this isn't explored further in the film. On three occasions, Tim clearly engages in pica: once by eating paint chips off of a green urn, another time by dipping his finger in a pail of paint, and finally by eating mud. He does this when no one is looking, so his family remains bewildered by his transient illnesses. At one point he becomes lethargic and seems ill enough to need medical attention, but Chris shrugs it off by saying that Tim always manages to get through these episodes on his own.

Child & Adolescent Psychiatric Disorders

TIC CODE, THE

Diagnosis Portrayed: Tourette's Disorder
DSM-IV-TR Code: 307.23

Accuracy Rating:
★★/★★★

Character's Name: Miles Caraday/Gregory Hines
Actor's Name: Christopher Marquette/Tyrone Pike

Signs & Symptoms: Motor tics (multiple)
Onset before age 18 years
Tics occur many times per day, nearly every day
Vocal tics (multiple)

Year of Release: 1999 **Country:** USA
Language: English **Genre:** Drama **Time:** 91 min.

Post Script:
Miles is a gifted pianist who longs to learn his craft by playing jazz. For a minor, he seems to get a lot of access to one particular night club before their shows and impresses the two bartenders with his skill. Miles gets a chance to play with one of his idols, sax man Pike. Anxiety provoking situations cause Miles to experience a worsening of his Tourette's disorder, which is manifested by both motor and vocal tics. Pike ostensibly suffers from the same condition, but in the context of the movie has learned to disguise his tics by, for example, pretending that he is coughing. Pike's role in the movie is a far less accurate depiction. The movie strays onto thinner ice by its shameless and unnecessary criticism of Kenny G (as if Pike's tics somehow prevented him from achieving similar status in the music world). Kenny G is an outstanding player, a generous and accessible celebrity, and such a class act that he wouldn't stoop to criticize someone else's creative efforts. He rocks!

Reel to Real: Psychiatric Conditions in Cinema

 LONELIEST RUNNER, THE

 Diagnosis Portrayed: Enuresis
DSM-IV-TR Code: 307.6

 Accuracy Rating:
★★★/★★★

 Character's Name: John Curtis
Actor's Name: Lance Kerwin/Michael Landon

 Signs & Symptoms:
Age is older than 5 years
Causes problems in social and academic functioning
Repeated voiding of urine into bed or clothes

 Year of Release: 1976 **Country:** USA
Language: English **Genre:** Drama **Time:** 74 min.

Post Script:
John is 13 and is stricken with enuresis. He has developed a new plan to hide it from his parents, which includes getting up early, changing his pyjamas and sheets, and going back to bed just before he is supposed to officially wake up. He then takes his soiled materials to a laundromat, using his lunch money and pilfered coins from his mother to pay for the washing and drying. His mother Alice (DeAnn Mears) thinks that her son is simply too lazy to get out of bed at night and sees his enuresis as a personal affront to her child-rearing abilities. When she finds out that John hasn't been able to remain dry at night, she punishes him by hanging his soiled sheets out of his bedroom window, forcing John to run home ahead of his school mates on a daily basis, which over time makes him a superb athlete. In addition to being an outstanding depiction of enuresis, Alice gives a very accurate portrayal of a paranoid personality disorder (see also page 66).

Child & Adolescent Psychiatric Disorders

SHINE

Diagnosis Portrayed: Encopresis
DSM-IV-TR Code: 307.7

Accuracy Rating:
★★★/★★★

Character's Name: David Helfgott (as an adolescent)
Actor's Name: Noah Taylor

Signs & Symptoms:
Age is older than 4 years
Causes problems in social and academic functioning
Passage of feces into inappropriate places

Year of Release: 1996 **Country:** Australia
Language: English **Genre:** Drama **Time:** 105 min.

Post Script:

This movie is also recommended for its accurate portrayal of schizoaffective disorder (see page 20). The main character, David Helfgott, is portrayed by three actors to cover different stages in his life. As an adolescent, David continues to wet the bed and in one scene, has an episode of encopresis in the bathtub. The diagnostic criteria allow for the passage of feces to be both involuntary and intentional. Prior to the episode shown in *Shine*, David had been experiencing increasing degrees of conflict with his father Peter (Armin Mueller-Stahl). David's talents as a pianist garner international attention, and it becomes clear that David will need to leave Australia on a music scholarship. Peter lost most of his family of origin to concentration camps in W.W. II, and is dogmatic about keeping his family together (giving an excellent portrayal of paranoid personality disorder — p. 66). Despite the clear detrimental effect on David's career, Peter's attempts to control the family escalate in direct proportion to David's reputation as a pianist.

Reel to Real: Psychiatric Conditions in Cinema

QUIET ROOM, THE

Diagnosis Portrayed: Selective Mutism
DSM-IV-TR Code: 313.23

Accuracy Rating:
★★★/★★★

Character's Name: Unnamed in this movie
Actor's Name: Phoebe Ferguson and Chloe Ferguson

Signs & Symptoms:
Adequate language skills are present
Failure to speak in social situations
Social function is interfered with
Speaks in situations other than the ones that cause the difficulty

Year of Release: 1996 **Country:** Australia/Italy/France
Language: English **Genre:** Drama **Time:** 92 min.

PostScript:
The unnamed main character in this film is seen in two time periods, roughly as a three-year-old and a seven-year-old. Her life at the earlier age is quite happy. There is lots of loving interaction with her parents and she is allowed to do her favorite thing, which is to sleep between them in their bed. Parental discord, called "sharpness" in the movie is the reason that she stops speaking to them at the later age. It becomes a silent protest to their heated exchanges and continual vacillation about dissolving the marriage. The girl has acquired excellent language skills prior to the selective mutism, and does sporadically speak, though not to her parents until quite late in the film. There is a narration track so the audience is party to the girl's thoughts, which contain a mixture of humor, sarcasm, advice, hope, and despair. The film is also an excellent example of the value of art therapy in reaching people, as the girl portrays her difficulties in this medium very clearly.

Cognitive Disorders

SNOWS OF KILIMANJARO, THE

Diagnosis Portrayed: Delirium
DSM-IV-TR Code: 293.0

Accuracy Rating:
★★/★★★

Character's Name: Harry Street
Actor's Name: Gregory Peck

Signs & Symptoms:
Changes in cognition
Fluctuating level of consciousness
Physiological evidence of a general medical condition causing the disturbance
Rapid development of symptoms

Year of Release: 1952 **Country:** USA
Language: English **Genre:** Drama **Time:** 114 min.

PostScript:
Street gets a serious infection from a thorn scratch while on an African safari and becomes delirious as a result. The timing of the infection and Street's physiological changes (sweating, restlessness, fluctuating level of consciousness, and malaise) are all clearly related. As Street succumbs to the delirium, he reviews many significant events from his life and verbalizes them while being cared for by his wife, Helen (Susan Hayward). Unfortunately, the great love of Street's life, Cynthia Green (Ava Gardner) features prominently in his reminiscences, as do his exploits with Countess Liz (Hildegard Neff). The depiction would have been more accurate if Street had shown signs of disorientation, perceptual disturbances (such as hallucinations), and language disturbances instead of just having the flashbacks, which are presumed to be accurate and not figments of his imagination.

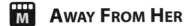

Away From Her

Diagnosis Portrayed: Dementia of the Alzheimer's Type
DSM-IV-TR Code: 294.10

Accuracy Rating:
★★★/★★★

Character's Name: Fiona Anderson
Actor's Name: Julie Christie

Signs & Symptoms:
Agnosia (failure to recognize husband)
Executive functioning impairment
Gradual onset of symptoms
Memory impairment
Significant difficulties in social or occupational functioning

Year of Release: 2006 **Country:** Canada
Language: English **Genre:** Drama **Time:** 110 min.

PostScript:
At the beginning of the film, Fiona has already developed a dementing illness and is slowly declining in her level of function. She puts a frying pan in the freezer instead of in the cupboard, but shortly afterwards her memory loss becomes more serious. During a solo cross-country skiing jaunt, she becomes lost and simply waits on a bridge for something to happen instead of asking for assistance. Fiona and her husband Grant (Gordon Pinsent) face the heart-wrenching but inevitable decision to have her placed in a long-term care facility. New residents are faced with a thirty-day period where they cannot receive visitors and Grant hasn't been apart from Fiona for this long in 44 years. In the month that follows, Fiona entirely forgets about Grant and doesn't recognize his face when he comes to see her. Repeated attempts on his part do not invoke the desired memories.

Cognitive Disorders

 # Aurora Borealis

 Diagnosis Portrayed: Dementia Due to Parkinson's Disease
DSM-IV-TR Code: 294.11

 Accuracy Rating:
★★★/★★★

 Character's Name: Ronald Shorter
Actor's Name: Donald Sutherland

 Signs & Symptoms:
Akinesia (slowed movements)
Depressed mood
Disinhibition (behavioral problems)
Disturbances in executive functioning
Memory impairment
Postural instability
Tremor

 Year of Release: 2005 **Country:** USA/Canada
Language: English **Genre:** Drama **Time:** 110 min.

PostScript:
Shorter suffers from a rapidly progressive course of this illness, and the main features of dementia and his movement disorder are portrayed very well. The main features of Parkinson's disease are evident the first time we see him — tremor, rigidity and postural problems. He still has a wide range of facial expression, so the masked facies isn't prominent. The script in the movie doesn't seem to account for the possibility that dementia can occur as a consequence of Parkinson's disease, since in one scene Shorter's home-care clinician Kate (Juliette Lewis) is concerned that he may develop co-morbid Alzheimer's disease (referred to here as the "A-bomb"). Shorter also displays several symptoms of depression, which is a common consequence of this disorder.

Reel to Real: Psychiatric Conditions in Cinema

MEMENTO

Diagnosis Portrayed: Amnestic Disorder
DSM-IV-TR Code: 294.0

Accuracy Rating:
★★★/★★★

Character's Name: Leonard Shelby
Actor's Name: Guy Pearce

Signs & Symptoms:
Memory impairment: inability to learn new information
Significant impairment in social and occupational functioning
Trauma was the cause of amnesia

Year of Release: 2000 **Country:** USA
Language: English **Genre:** Mystery **Time:** 113 min.

PostScript:
Shelby develops anterograde amnesia after experiencing a head injury while trying to fend off his attackers in a home invasion. Shelby's wife is sexually assaulted and murdered, and he devotes his life to trying to find the responsible parties. Unfortunately, Shelby is unable to retain new memories for more that a few minutes, so he tries to piece things together with notes, photographs, and by tattooing himself with important developments in what be believes to be the sequence of events. Shelby's condition is exploited by two shady characters Natalie (Carrie-Anne Moss) and Teddy (Joe Pantoliano), who conscript the unwitting Shelby into doing some of their dirty work. *Memento* received widespread acclaim for the accuracy of the memory disturbance portrayed and the resulting disability. The film is not shown in a linear sequence, making for an engaging viewing experience in trying to figure out exactly what happened.

Substance-Related Disorders

AFFLICTION

Diagnosis Portrayed: Alcohol Dependence
DSM-IV-TR Code: 303.90

Accuracy Rating:
★★★/★★★

Character's Name: Glen Whitehouse
Actor's Name: James Coburn

Signs & Symptoms:
Alcohol use that is heavy and prolonged
Consumption continues despite social and occupational consequences
Substantial amount of time spent in obtaining and consuming alcohol
Tolerance to alcohol intake

Year of Release: 1997 **Country:** USA
Language: English **Genre:** Drama **Time:** 114 min.

PostScript:

The "affliction" referred to in this movie is the double curse of alcohol dependence and physical abuse. Whitehouse is a menacing bear of a man who is inebriated during the whole film, as well as in various flashbacks. When we first see him, he is sitting in his living room in a stuporous state with his front door open in the middle of a New Hampshire winter. His wife has frozen to death upstairs, but when he tries to rouse her, he doesn't even notice that she has passed away. Later at her funeral he has been drinking again and demonstrates many signs of alcohol intoxication, including: slurred speech, incoordination, unsteady gait, and labile mood. His impaired judgment and inappropriate aggressive behavior in the funeral scene are particularly well portrayed as Whitehouse tries to become violent when giving a tribute to his wife and has to be restrained by one of his sons.

Reel to Real: Psychiatric Conditions in Cinema

HOOSIERS

Diagnosis Portrayed: Alcohol Intoxication and Alcohol Withdrawal
DSM-IV-TR Code: 303.00 and 291.81

Accuracy Rating:
★★★/★★★

Character's Name: Shooter Flatch
Actor's Name: Dennis Hopper

Signs & Symptoms:
Agitation (intoxication)
Anxiety (withdrawal)
Attention is impaired (intoxication)
Incoordination (intoxication)
Slurred speech (intoxication)
Tremor (withdrawal)
Unsteady gait (intoxication)

Year of Release: 1986 **Country:** USA
Language: English **Genre:** Drama **Time:** 114 min.

PostScript:
Shooter is the town drunk in this story about a 1950's Indiana basketball team that wins the State championship. He is a keen observer of the game and the proud father of one of the players. He is offered the position of assistant coach if he can remain sober. Shooter agrees, but shows up inebriated at one game and stumbles right onto the court. Other signs of intoxication portrayed in this scene are slurred speech, incoordination, and impaired judgment. Shooter finally agrees to give up drinking and is admitted to the local hospital. Here, he goes into alcohol withdrawal and is shown to be anxious, agitated, sweating, and tremulous. Later, he describes transient hallucinations ("bad visions") but does not go on to have an alcohol withdrawal delirium.

Substance-Related Disorders

 # DAYS OF WINE AND ROSES

 Diagnosis Portrayed: Alcohol Withdrawal Delirium
DSM-IV-TR Code: 291.0

 Accuracy Rating:
★★★/★★★

 Character's Name: Joe Clay
Actor's Name: Jack Lemmon

 Signs & Symptoms:
Cognitive deficits
Fluctuating level of consciousness
Perceptual abnormalities
Rapid onset of symptoms
Symptoms related to the abrupt cessation of alcohol

 Year of Release: 1962 **Country:** USA
Language: English **Genre:** Romance **Time:** 117 min.

PostScript:
Clay works in public relations and often socializes with his clients. At the beginning of the film, he is a "functional alcoholic" who still manages in social and occupational roles. Joe meets Kirsten Arnesen (Lee Remick), who soon replaces her fondness for chocolate with an addiction to alcohol. After losing a series of jobs, Clay realizes that his drinking is beyond his ability to control. He manages to avoid alcohol for several weeks but then goes on a bender and ends up in the violent ward of a psychiatric hospital going through delirium tremens (DTs). Here, Joe can be seen sweating and writhing on the floor in a highly agitated state. He experiences perceptual abnormalities that cause him to be absolutely terrified of the hospital staff when they come to check on him. He is so disoriented and confused that he requires a straitjacket so that he doesn't hurt himself or anyone else.

Reel to Real: Psychiatric Conditions in Cinema

REQUIEM FOR A DREAM

Diagnosis Portrayed: Amphetamine Intoxication With Perceptual Disturbances
DSM-IV-TR Code: 292.89

Accuracy Rating:
★★★/★★★

Character's Name: Sara Goldfarb
Actor's Name: Ellen Burstyn

Signs & Symptoms: Agitation and restlessness
Autonomic dysregulation
Hallucinatory experiences
Weight loss

Year of Release: 2000 **Country:** USA
Language: English **Genre:** Romance **Time:** 102 min.

PostScript:
Sara is a lonely widow who gets invited to be part of the audience for a TV show. This opportunity rallies her and in a short time becomes the focus of her life. She envisions herself becoming a featured guest, and decides that she should lose weight before her appearance. Sara tries dieting but is tormented by continual cravings. On the recommendation of a friend, she attends a diet clinic and receives a prescription for amphetamines. Sara is soon full of vitality. Her appetite is suppressed and she loses weight effortlessly. She has energy and radiates confidence. In the scene where her son returns to tell her he is buying her a television set, Sara is euphoric, talkative, and restless. Because the medications are prescribed, Sara ignores the warning and continues to take the amphetamines in increased amounts because they eventually stop having the same effect on her appetite. When she increases her dose, Sara develops perceptual disturbances.

Substance-Related Disorders

SIXTY CUPS OF COFFEE

Diagnosis Portrayed: Caffeine Intoxication
DSM-IV-TR Code: 305.90

Accuracy Rating:
★★★/★★★

Character's Name: Rickie Cass
Actor's Name: Jerry Broome

Signs & Symptoms:
Agitation
Diuresis
Muscle twitching
Nervousness
Restlessness

Year of Release: 2000 **Country:** USA
Language: English **Genre:** Short **Time:** 8 min.

PostScript:
The protagonist in this short wonders if 60 cups (the rumored daily intake of Honoré de Balzac) of coffee can kill a man. For no apparent reason other than to give it a try, he enters a diner and proceeds to drink cup after cup (later pot after pot) to see what will happen. The indifferent waitress (Kelley West) becomes concerned when she learns the extent of Cass' plan and that she might be liable for anything that happens to him. Two patrons in the diner place bets on Cass, and a horrified (but oddly intrigued) mother watches on with her son. Cass starts to develop symptoms of intoxication, including periods of confusion. This short is available for viewing at: www.openfilm.com/videos/sixty_cups_of_coffee

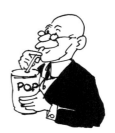

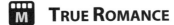

True Romance

Diagnosis Portrayed: Cannabis Intoxication
DSM-IV-TR Code: 292.89

Accuracy Rating:
★★★/★★★

Character's Name: Floyd
Actor's Name: Brad Pitt

Signs & Symptoms:
Appetite increase
Confusion/disorientation
Euphoria
Impaired judgment
Memory impairment
Social withdrawal

Year of Release: 1993 **Country:** USA
Language: English **Genre:** Action **Time:** 120 min.

PostScript:
Floyd's role in the movie is one of the secondary characters. He is stoned the whole movie, rarely even getting off the couch. Floyd demonstrates impaired judgment by giving the motel address of an out-of-town friend to Virgil (James Gandolfini), an organized crime hit man without even asking why he would be looking for this person. Floyd feels that Virgil was condescending towards him and challenges Virgil to a fight, but this is after Virgil has already left. Floyd is at times edgy, particularly when people do things around him that he has trouble keeping up with because of his state of intoxication (e.g. someone taking a phone of out his hands). In another scene, Floyd is confronted by four men openly brandishing a wide array of firearms, and he doesn't seem to even take notice of them. He tries to give them directions to another motel, but is too stoned to orient himself properly.

Substance-Related Disorders

BLOW

Diagnosis Portrayed: Cocaine Abuse
DSM-IV-TR Code: 305.60

Accuracy Rating:
★★★/★★★

Character's Name: George Jung/Mirtha Jung
Actor's Name: Johnny Depp/Penélope Cruz

Signs & Symptoms:
Anxiety/psychomotor agitation
Cardiac problems
Euphoria
Hypervigilance
Impaired judgment
Mood lability
Weight loss

Year of Release: 2001 **Country:** USA
Language: English **Genre:** Biography **Time:** 124 min.

PostScript:
For much of this film, the effects of cocaine are eclipsed by the lifestyle aspects of the drug trade. When Jung watches the birth of his daughter, he collapses in the delivery room because of the cardiac complications of cocaine. Prior to his collapse, we see him making involuntary movements (particularly his right arm and hand). He also doesn't have his surgical mask on and appears to be confused. Some of the more flagrant psychological effects of cocaine are portrayed by his wife Mirtha. Though she is a dramatic and impulsive person to begin with, she becomes reckless, destructive, and unable to control herself. The scene where she nearly causes a car crash in front of a police cruiser is a particularly good example of the mood lability, impaired judgment, and instantaneous anger that is seen with cocaine abuse.

Reel to Real: Psychiatric Conditions in Cinema

SCARFACE

Diagnosis Portrayed: Cocaine Intoxication
DSM-IV-TR Code: 292.89

Accuracy Rating:
★★★/★★★

Character's Name: Tony Montana
Actor's Name: Al Pacino

Signs & Symptoms:
Confusion/disorganization
Euphoria
Hypervigilance/suspiciousness
Mood lability
Perspiration
Weight loss

Year of Release: 1983 **Country:** USA
Language: English **Genre:** Crime **Time:** 170 min.

PostScript:
Montana is a Cuban refugee who, through a blend of ruthlessness and cunning, establishes himself as a top-level cocaine dealer. As the movie progresses, both Montana and his wife Elvira (Michelle Pfeiffer) use increasing amounts of cocaine. Elvira seems to use cocaine to control her appetite, but does not display many of the signs of acute intoxication. Montana becomes increasingly erratic as he consumes larger and larger amounts. He becomes hypervigilant and suspicious of everyone. Montana kills his long-time associate Manny (Steven Bauer), double crosses his Bolivian supplier, and becomes increasingly confused and disorganized due to cocaine use. In the action-packed final sequence of the film, Montana snorts a considerable amount of cocaine, which causes him to sweat profusely and become irritable and increasingly tense.

Substance-Related Disorders

Fear And Loathing in Las Vegas

Diagnosis Portrayed: Hallucinogen Intoxication
DSM-IV-TR Code: 292.89

Accuracy Rating:
★★★/★★★

Character's Name: Raoul Duke/Dr. Gonzo
Actor's Name: Johnny Depp/Benicio Del Toro

Signs & Symptoms:	Blurred vision
	Impaired judgment
	Incoordination
	Mood lability
	Palpitations
	Sweating

Year of Release: 1998 **Country:** USA
Language: English   **Genre:** Comedy **Time:** 118 min.

PostScript:
Duke has the trunk in his convertible loaded with most types of abusable substances, but appears to be under the influence of LSD ("blotter acid") at the beginning of the film and then takes another hit as he is driving. In every scene in this movie the two main characters are under the influence of mind-altering substances. The first effect of LSD that Duke experiences is the visual hallucination of bats swarming around him. He becomes quite agitated and stops the car to let Gonzo drive. They pick up a hitchhiker (Tobey Maguire), and it is here that Duke's aberrant thought processes are clearly portrayed. Duke is quite paranoid that the hitchhiker will seek out the police as soon as possible, illustrating thoughts of persecution. Duke displays impaired judgment repeatedly by driving recklessly, brandishing firearms, leaving restaurants without paying, etc.

Reel to Real: **Psychiatric Conditions in Cinema**

 # BASKETBALL DIARIES, THE

 Diagnosis Portrayed: Inhalant Intoxication
DSM-IV-TR Code: 292.89

 Accuracy Rating:
★★★/★★★

 Character's Name: Jim Carroll
Actor's Name: Leonardo DiCaprio

 Signs & Symptoms:
Blurred vision/diplopia
Euphoria
Incoordination
Lethargy
Slurred speech
Unsteady gait

 Year of Release: 1995 **Country:** USA
Language: English **Genre:** Action **Time:** 102 min.

PostScript:
In the first couple of minutes of the film, Carroll and his friends board the Staten Island Ferry and use an inhalant. They pour a yellowish liquid onto a rag and in turn hold it over their mouths and noses. Unfortunately for the sake of this portrayal, Pedro (James Madio) is overcome by the fumes and vomits on another passenger named Vinnie (Vincent Pastore). Vinnie gives chase and the full effects of the inhalant aren't depicted in this scene. Mickey (Mark Wahlberg) later reads from Carroll's diary about one of their huffing episodes. They were inhaling carbolic cleaning fluid. After 4 deep inhalations, Carroll felt as if he was "*sailing someplace else with little bells ringing in his ears.*" He also describes a vision in which he was paddling a "*canoe on black water that was flowing backwards,*" and that he saw in the clouds "*spooky funhouse faces that were laughing at him.*"

Substance-Related Disorders

 # No Smoking

 Diagnosis Portrayed: Nicotine Withdrawal
DSM-IV-TR Code: 292.0

Accuracy Rating:
★★★/★★★

 Character's Name: Goofy
Actor's Name: Pinto Colvig (voice)

 Signs & Symptoms:
Abrupt cessation of nicotine
Difficulty concentrating
Dysphoric mood
Irritability
Restlessness

 Year of Release: 1951 **Country:** USA
Language: English **Genre:** Animated **Time:** 6 min.

PostScript:
Goofy (listed in this cartoon as George Geef) smokes constantly. He lights up first thing in the morning, smokes at work, and needs one last coffin nail before he goes to bed. He tries to quit, and goes through a number of withdrawal symptoms that are accurately portrayed, including the minute-to-minute struggle that most smokers face when they try to give up this habit. The withdrawal symptoms test Goofy to his limits. Goofy is finally able to kick his habit, but it takes a fairly extreme measure to bring this about. Included in this cartoon is a brief history of smoking, with various versions of Goofy playing prominent people (such as Christopher Columbus). There are also several parodies of major cigarette brands. There is an interesting segment where a desperate Goofy lists off common slang terms for cigarettes, which includes "fag" — a term usually used in the UK and Australia, and "weed," which now of course "reefers" to marijuana.

Reel to Real: **Psychiatric Conditions in Cinema**

M BASQUIAT

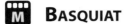

Dx **Diagnosis Portrayed:** Opioid Intoxication
DSM-IV-TR Code: 292.89

★ **Accuracy Rating:**
★★★/★★★

C **Character's Name:** Jean Michel Basquiat
Actor's Name: Jeffrey Wright

Sx **Signs & Symptoms:**
Decreased attention span
Drowsiness
Euphoria
Nodding head

I **Year of Release:** 1996 **Country:** USA
Language: English   **Genre:** Biography **Time:** 96 min.

PostScript:
Basquiat was a New York City artist who initially gained recognition for his graffiti. As his fame and income grew, so did his drug use. There is one scene in particular that contains a very accurate portrayal of opioid intoxication. Morpheus was the Greek God of dreams, and it is his name from which the word morphine is derived. After using heroin, Basquiat is seen to be in a hypnotic state staring at a sheet of canvas that covers his floor. He starts imagining that he sees a growing stack of car tires on the canvas. When it gets to a certain height, he smears part of the tread with white paint. Basquiat seems both pleased and amused by his drug-induced vision, which is an example of the euphoria that accompanies opioid use. He seems rather drowsy after using the heroin, and has difficulty sustaining his attention. His head keeps nodding up and down, which is called "being on the nod." Basquiat is revived from this trip by his girlfriend Gina (Claire Forlani), who pounds on his chest until he regains full consciousness.

Substance-Related Disorders

 # BASKETBALL DIARIES, THE

 Diagnosis Portrayed: Opioid Withdrawal
DSM-IV-TR Code: 292.0

 Accuracy Rating:
★★★/★★★

 Character's Name: Jim Carroll
Actor's Name: Leonardo DiCaprio

 Signs & Symptoms:
Dysphoric mood
Insomnia
Muscle and joint pain
Rhinorrhea/runny nose

 Year of Release: 1995 **Country:** USA
Language: English **Genre:** Action **Time:** 102 min.

PostScript:
Carroll turns to a life of crime to support his heroin addiction. All of his time is taken up obtaining money to buy heroin or being under its influence. He shares needles with others. He sleeps on the street and lives in derelict housing with other addicts. In addition to becoming a car thief and burglar, he becomes a sex trade worker to support his habit. Yet nothing seems to pull him out of his addiction. One heroin trip leaves Carroll unconscious in the snow, and it is by mere chance that he is found by his friend Reggie (Ernie Hudson). Carroll soon goes into opioid withdrawal, which the movie accurately portrays. The depiction of opioid use in this film is particularly good because it isn't glamorized. Carroll loses everything after becoming a heroin addict — his education, his friends, his mother, his dignity, his health, and very nearly his life (on several occasions). He is utterly unable to stop on his own, and it is only after being incarcerated that he gets the opportunity and perspective to give up his addiction.

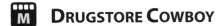

Drugstore Cowboy

Diagnosis Portrayed: Opioid Abuse
DSM-IV-TR Code: 305.50

Accuracy Rating:
★★★/★★★

Character's Name: Bob
Actor's Name: Matt Dillon

Signs & Symptoms:
Drug use in physically hazardous situations
Legal problems
Recurrent drug use causing failure to fulfil major obligations
Substance use causing social and interpersonal problems

Year of Release: 1989 **Country:** USA
Language: English **Genre:** Action **Time:** 102 min.

PostScript:

Bob explains to an intake coordinator at a methadone clinic why he feels harassed by her questions: *"I'm a junkie. I like drugs. I like the whole lifestyle, but it just didn't pay off. You know, you don't see my kind of people, because my kind of people don't come down here and beg dope. They go out and get it. And if they miss, they go to jail and they kick along with nothing in some holding tank."* When asked if he would be interested in becoming an addiction counselor, Bob scoffs at the idea and offers the following explanation: *"To begin with, nobody, and I mean nobody can talk a junkie out of using. You can talk to them for years, but sooner or later they're going to get a hold of something. Maybe it's not dope, maybe it's booze, maybe it's glue, maybe its gasoline. Maybe it's a gunshot in the head."*

Substance-Related Disorders

 # I'M DANCING AS FAST AS I CAN

 Diagnosis Portrayed: Sedative, Hypnotic or Anxiolytic Dependence
DSM-IV-TR Code: 304.10

 Accuracy Rating:
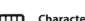

Character's Name: Barbara Gordon
Actor's Name: Jill Clayburgh

 Signs & Symptoms:
Efforts to cut down are unsuccessful
Physiological dependence
Substance taken in larger amounts than originally intended
Tolerance to the effects of the drug
Use continues despite problems

 Year of Release: 1982 **Country:** USA
Language: English **Genre:** Drama **Time:** 107 min.

PostScript:
Barbara is a successful TV producer who runs on nerves and nicotine, and is benzodiazepine dependent, popping pills whenever she feels slightly anxious. She has a bottle on her table at work and tablets hidden in her cigarette package. Barbara has bags of pills stashed in many hiding places in her apartment. Prior to going to a ceremony where she is nominated for (and wins) an award, she sews a small sac into her dress that contains two pills. She demonstrates some of the signs of benzodiazepine intoxication during her acceptance speech. Her memory is impaired and her thoughts are not fluent. After leaving the stage, she struggles momentarily with one of the assistants who reaches for the award because Barbara forgets that they are props and that the real one will be sent to her when after it is engraved.

Reel to Real: **Psychiatric Conditions in Cinema**

 # I'm Dancing as Fast as I Can

 Diagnosis Portrayed: Sedative, Hypnotic or Anxiolytic Withdrawal
DSM-IV-TR Code: 292.0

 Accuracy Rating:
★★★ / ★★★

 Character's Name: Barbara Gordon
Actor's Name: Jill Clayburgh

 Signs & Symptoms:
Agitation
Anxiety
Insomnia
Seizures
Tremor

 Year of Release: 1982 **Country:** USA
Language: English **Genre:** Drama **Time:** 107 min.

PostScript:
Later on in the film as Barbara is repeatedly made aware of the problems her benzodiazepine use is causing for her, she decides to abruptly quit taking Valium® and hangs up on her psychiatrist before he can explain the risks she faces. For the first several hours she feels fine because Valium® has a long duration of action. Later she clearly develops benzodiazepine withdrawal, shown by a number of accurate symptoms. In the scene on the beach, Barbara has a generalized seizure, which is a serious complication of benzodiazepine withdrawal. She develops a serious craving for more Valium® and tries to surreptitiously order more from a pharmacy. The tag line for this film nicely summarizes Barbara's dependence on benzodiazepines — "Two In The Morning. Two Before Lunch. Two After Dinner. Two Before Bed. Every Day."

Medical Conditions Causing Psychiatric Disorders

JESUS OF MONTREAL

Diagnosis Portrayed: Psychotic Disorder Due to a Head Injury
DSM-IV-TR Code: 293.81

Accuracy Rating:
★★/★★★

Character's Name: Daniel Coulombe
Actor's Name: Lothaire Bluteau

Signs & Symptoms: Delusional beliefs
Head injury

Year of Release: 1989 **Country:** Canada/France
Language: French **Genre:** Drama **Time:** 118 min.

PostScript:
Coulombe is hired by a church to revamp the Passion Play, the crucifixion of Christ, for a summer theater. The production is an instant hit but the troupe's new content displeases the religious authorities and they shut down the play. Without permission, the actors begin one last performance and a scuffle ensues, knocking Coulombe, who had been playing Jesus, to the ground from his cross. He sustains a head injury and loses consciousness. He awakens in the ER and decides to leave. A blood vessel has ruptured in his brain and for the last half hour of his life, Coulombe seems to believe that he is Jesus and offers guidance to people walking by him in a subway station. Many of the statements he makes are similar to the lines he had in the play. While no one actually asks him to identify himself, his demeanor after the head injury is quite different from his usual personality. It seems reasonable to assume that if he had been asked who he was, he may well have said Jesus, and if so, this would be a delusion, qualifying him for the diagnosis of psychotic disorder due to a head injury.

Reel to Real: Psychiatric Conditions in Cinema

LORENZO'S OIL

Diagnosis Portrayed: Dementia Due to a Metabolic Abnormality
DSM-IV-TR Code: 294.81

Accuracy Rating:
★★★/★★★

Character's Name: Lorenzo Odone
Actor's Name: Various

Signs & Symptoms: Behavioral disturbances
Emotional lability
Intellectual decline

Year of Release: 1992 **Country:** USA
Language: English **Genre:** Drama **Time:** 129 min.

PostScript:
This is a heart-wrenching movie based on a true story. Lorenzo (played by a variety of actors) is a bright, healthy five year-old boy who among other things speaks three languages. His father works for the World Bank and after spending three years in Africa, Lorenzo and his family return home. Within a short period of time Lorenzo develops an increasing number of behavior problems. He has angry outbursts, becomes hyperactive and inattentive, and is moody. Lorenzo's teachers cannot handle these disruptions and want him placed in a special education class. Lorenzo has a thorough medical investigation and is found to have a rare inherited metabolic abnormality called adrenoleukodystrophy (ALD). This progressive condition kills brain cells, leading to dementia and a wide range of physical complications. As his ALD progresses Lorenzo becomes withdrawn, forgetful, emotionally labile, and develops a number of neurological deficits, all of which are due to loss of brain function secondary to his metabolic abnormality.

Medical Conditions Causing Psychiatric Disorders

REGARDING HENRY

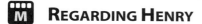

Diagnosis Portrayed: Amnestic Disorder and Personality Change Due to Anoxia
DSM-IV-TR Code: 294.0 and 310.1

Accuracy Rating:
★★★/★★★

Character's Name: Henry Turner
Actor's Name: Harrison Ford

Signs & Symptoms:
Agnosia (problems in identifying things)
Aphasia (language disturbance)
Disturbances in executive functioning
Memory impairment for events prior to the trauma
Personality changes (permanent)

Year of Release: 1991 **Country:** USA
Language: English **Genre:** Drama **Time:** 108 min.

PostScript:
Turner, a hard-charging, successful lawyer, is the picture of compassion during a big case but is arrogant, dictatorial, and selfish socially. Proving that smoking can indeed be a health hazard, Turner tries to buy cigarettes from a convenience store that is being robbed. The nervous gunman shoots Turner twice — once in the right side of the head and the other in the left side of his chest. Surprisingly it is the chest wound that causes the most damage. The bullet hits a major vessel and the blood loss is so severe that his brain is deprived of oxygen (anoxia) and is permanently damaged. Turner undergoes a lengthy physical and mental rehabilitation. At first he is mute but later recovers his speech. He has significant memory gaps, forgetting even his own daughter. He needs to be reminded how to tie his shoelaces, read, etc.

Reel to Real: Psychiatric Conditions in Cinema

 # Madness Of King George, The

 Diagnosis Portrayed: Mood Disorder Due to Porphyria
DSM-IV-TR Code: 293.83

 Accuracy Rating:
★★★/★★★

 Character's Name: King George III
Actor's Name: Nigel Hawthorne

 Signs & Symptoms: Evidence of porphyria (dark urine)
Hypomanic/manic symptoms

 Year of Release: 1994 **Country:** UK
Language: English **Genre:** Biography **Time:** 107 min.

PostScript:
King George has psychiatric difficulties that are apparent from the beginning of the film. He is boisterous, disinhibited, and distractible. When he encounters a pig farm and a game of cricket, he cannot help but energetically throw himself into the action. King George is perpetually rushing and speaks rapidly to those around him. He ravishes an attractive noblewoman in front of the Queen and other members of his entourage. His mood, while generally jovial, is labile. He has several angry outbursts. In one scene the king speaks in rhymes. He has difficulty restraining his impulses and at times his behavior becomes outlandish and is an embarrassment to the country. In the portrayal shown in this movie, King George has signs and symptoms that are consistent with the hypomanic phase, and later the manic phase of bipolar disorder. King George's physical ailment is a matter of speculation but is noted at the end of the film to be porphyria. King George is depicted as suffering from severe intermittent abdominal pain and constipation, both of which are consistent with porphyria. Other common psychiatric complications include depression and psychosis.

Medical Conditions Causing Psychiatric Disorders

BIGGER THAN LIFE

Diagnosis Portrayed: Corticosteroid-Induced Mood Disorder, With Manic Features, With Onset During Intoxication
DSM-IV-TR Code: 292.84

Accuracy Rating:
★★★/★★★

Character's Name: Ed Avery
Actor's Name: James Mason

Signs & Symptoms:
Corticosteroid use is etiologically related to the onset of the symptoms
Decreased need for sleep
Delusions of persecution
Elevated and irritable mood
Grandiosity
Mood lability

Year of Release: 1956 **Country:** USA
Language: English **Genre:** Drama **Time:** 95 min.

PostScript:
Avery is a dedicated teacher, father, and husband. He has paroxysmal attacks that are eventually diagnosed as periarteritis nodosa, for which he is prescribed a corticosteroid. The medication significantly reduces his symptoms, but he starts to take it more often than it is prescribed. Avery's mood progresses through being elated to irritable, and he develops hypomania, then mania, and finally becomes frankly psychotic. As his mood escalates, he becomes increasingly talkative, opinionated, and demeaning. The movie reaches a chilling climax when Avery's son tries to hide the pill bottle from him. Avery predicts that his son will lead a life of crime and that he should, on moral grounds, kill him.

Reel to Real: Psychiatric Conditions in Cinema

AWAKENINGS

Diagnosis Portrayed: Catatonic Disorder Due to Encephalitis
DSM-IV-TR Code: 293.89

Accuracy Rating:
★★★/★★★

Character's Name: Lucy Fishman
Actor's Name: Alice Drummond

Signs & Symptoms:
Mutism
Negativism (automatic opposition)
Odd postures
Unresponsive to the environment

Year of Release: 1990 **Country:** USA
Language: English   **Genre:** Drama **Time:** 121 min.

PostScript:
Dr. Sayer (Robin Williams) is a researcher who agrees to work in a chronic care hospital. The particular ward where Sayer is assigned is occupied by patients that have either psychiatric or neurologic difficulties. Dr. Sayer rediscovers that five inpatients suffer from a post-encephalitic syndrome. The first patient shown with this condition is Lucy, who is mute and unresponsive to her surroundings. The odd postures she adopts are a good example of some of the movement abnormalities seen in catatonia. Later, she exhibits negativism when Dr. Sayer tries to help her towards a water fountain. Very good depictions of catatonic behavior can be seen in the old film clip shown by Dr. Peter Ingham (Max von Sydow). Patients seen in the hallways of the chronic ward can be seen engaging in repetitive activities such as rocking or grimacing that also constitute some of the behavior changes seen in a variety of serious mental illnesses.

Movie Index

Movie Name	Section	Page

A

A Fish Called Wanda	Child Psychiatry	80
A Secret Between Friends	Eating Disorders	55
A Streetcar Named Desire	Personality Disorders	71
Adventures of Priscilla, Queen of the Desert, The	Gender Identity Disorders	53
Affliction	Substance-Related Disorders	95
Aliens	Sleep Disorders	59
Analyze This	Anxiety Disorders	35
Annie Hall	Anxiety Disorders	39
Aurora Borealis	Cognitive Disorders	93
Awakenings	Medical Disorders	116
Away From Her	Cognitive Disorders	92

B

Backdraft	Impulse-Control Disorders	64
Bandits	Somatoform Disorders	43
Basketball Diaries, The	Substance-Related Disorders	104, 107
Basquiat	Substance-Related Disorders	106
Bell Jar, The	Psychotic Disorders	19
Best Little Girl in the World, The	Eating Disorders	54
Bigger Than Life	Medical Conditions	115
Blow	Substance-Related Disorders	101
Blue Velvet	Sexual Disorders	50
Bug	Psychotic Disorders	25
Bulworth	Sleep Disorders	56

C

Caine Mutiny, The	Personality Disorders	66
Canvas	Psychotic Disorders	17
Clean, Shaven	Psychotic Disorders	18
Copycat	Anxiety Disorders	36

Reel to Real: Psychiatric Conditions in Cinema

D

Days of Wine and Roses	Substance-Related Disorders	97
Defending Your Life	Anxiety Disorders	41
Delicate Art of Parking, The	Personality Disorders	74
Dirty, Filthy Love	Impulse-Control Disorders	65
Don't Say A Word	Factitious Disorder	45
Donnie Darko	Sleep Disorders	60
Drugstore Cowboy	Substance-Related Disorders	108

F

Fear and Loathing in Las Vegas	Substance-Related Disorders	103
Female Perversions	Impulse-Control Disorders	62

G

Good Son, The	Child Psychiatry	84

H

Hannah and Her Sisters	Somatoform Disorders	42
He Loves Me… He Loves Me Not	Psychotic Disorders	21
Heavenly Creatures	Psychotic Disorders	26
High Anxiety	Anxiety Disorders	40
Hoosiers	Substance-Related Disorders	96
Hospital, The	Mood Disorders	30
Hours, The	Mood Disorders	28

I

I'm Dancing as Fast as I Can	Substance-Related Disorders	109, 110
I Am Sam	Child Psychiatry	76
In Country	Anxiety Disorders	37
Insomnia	Sleep Disorders	58

Movie Index

Jesus of Montreal — Medical Conditions — 111
Just Like A Woman — Gender Identity Disorder — 51

Loneliest Runner, The — Child Psychiatry — 88
Lorenzo's Oil — Medical Conditions — 112

Mad Love — Mood Disorders — 34
Madness of King George, The — Medical Conditions — 114
Man Bites Dog — Personality Disorders — 69
Man Who Wasn't There, The — Personality Disorders — 67, 68
Matchstick Men — Anxiety Disorders — 38
Memento — Cognitive Disorders — 94
Michael Clayton — Mood Disorders — 33
Mr. Jones — Mood Disorders — 32
Mosquito Coast, The — Mood Disorders — 31
Mozart and the Whale — Child Psychiatry — 82
My Own Private Idaho — Sleep Disorders — 57

Nell — Child Psychiatry — 79
No Smoking — Substance-Related Disorders — 105
Nurse Betty — Dissociative Disorders — 48

Owning Mahowny — Impulse-Control Disorders — 63

Patch Adams — Mood Disorders — 29
Possessed — Psychotic Disorders — 16
Punch-Drunk Love — Impulse-Control Disorders — 61

Reel to Real: Psychiatric Conditions in Cinema

Q

Quiet Room, The	Child Psychiatry	90

R

Rain Man	Child Psychiatry	81
Red Dragon	Somatoform Disorders	44
Regarding Henry	Medical Conditions	113
Remains of the Day, The	Personality Disorders	75
Requiem for a Dream	Substance-Related Disorders	98
Royal Tenenbaums, The	Malingering	46

S

Scarface	Substance-Related Disorders	102
Secret, The	Child Psychiatry	78
Shine	Psychotic Disorders	20
Shine	Child Psychiatry	89
Single, White Female	Personality Disorders	70
Sixty Cups of Coffee	Substance-Related Disorders	99
Sliver	Sexual Disorder	52
Snake Pit, The	Psychotic Disorders	22
Snows of Kilimanjaro, The	Cognitive Disorders	91
Spider	Psychotic Disorders	15

T

Three Faces of Eve, The	Dissociative Disorders	47
Thumbsucker	Child Psychiatry	83
Tic Code, The	Child Psychiatry	87
True Romance	Substance-Related Disorders	100

U

Undertow	Child Psychiatry	86
Unfaithfully Yours	Psychotic Disorders	23
Unstrung Heroes	Psychotic Disorders	24

Movie Index

Wall Street	Personality Disorders	72
What's Eating Gilbert Grape	Child Psychiatry	77
Woodsman, The	Sexual Disorders	49
Wrong Man, The	Mood Disorders	27

Young Poisoner's Handbook, The	Child Psychiatry	85

Zelig	Personality Disorders	73

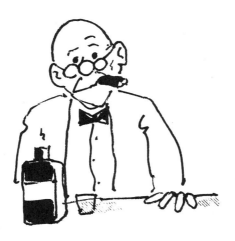

Reel to Real: Psychiatric Conditions in Cinema

All-Star Recommendations

Since the publication of *Reel Psychiatry* in 2003, I have constantly (and very happily) been discussing films and their educational role in psychiatry. I have frequently been asked about my favorite films, but they do not necessarily have content that is relevant to psychiatric educators. For the purpose of developing a "must have" list for teaching purposes, I have compiled a list movies here that I feel are of particular merit.

Memento, Wide Screen, Two-Disc Limited Edition

This movie is a masterpiece of filmmaking, intertwining an outstanding portrayal of amnestic disorder with a psychological thriller. The film is shown in alternating narratives, one in black-and-white (which are shown in chronological order), the other in color (shown in reverse chronological order). The main character is desperately trying to solve the murder of his wife, but lacks the ability to make new memories. Leads that he thinks are important to solving the case disappear in minutes. The special edition release of this film contains an audio commentary by the director Christopher Nolan and the original short story on which the story is based (*Memento Mori*) by his brother Jonathan. There is also a feature that allows you to watch the movie in its proper sequence. The Limited Edition DVD is packaged to look like a case file from a psychiatric institution, complete with hand-written notes. The DVD menus appear as if they are psychological tests, requiring that the viewer participate by choosing certain words, objects, and answers to play the movie or access special features.

Lars and the Real Girl

This movie is not included in this book, but is a very good portrayal of a young man (Lars, played by Ryan Gosling) who has prominent schizoid personality traits, though there are many confounding symptoms and behaviors that obscure the diagnosis. An article published by Dr. Norman Doidge on the movie *The English Patient* (Diagnosing the English Patient: Schizoid Fantasies of Being Skinless and of Being Buried Alive, J Am Psychoanal Assoc 2001; 49; 279) outlines many themes involving people with schizoid personalities that are present in this film. The other gem in this movie is the role of the family doctor/psychologist Dagmar (played by Patricia Clarkson). Though Lars is seemingly delusional, she masterfully develops a therapeutic alliance with him and helps to treat him without the use of medications or the need for hospitalization. Her immediate connection with his symptoms and education of the family are outstanding.

All-Star Movie Recommendations

Shine
This movie is a rare find. It traces the development of a serious mental disorder in a talented musician and shows him at three stages in his life. We get to see family dynamics compellingly displayed for us, trace how various characters seemingly make contributions to a self-fulfilling prophecy, and bear witness to the devastating effects of a psychotic disorder. The movie is that much more interesting because it is based on the life of David Helfgott, who still gives concerts. The movie is loaded with educational topics, including:
- Paranoid personality disorder (in the main character's father)
- Role of genetics in psychiatric disorders
- Enuresis and encopresis
- Health concerns in patients with chronic psychiatric illnesses
- The role of expressed emotion in family interactions
- Autonomy versus paternalism
- Diagnostic challenges
- Prodromal and residual symptoms in psychotic disorders
- Stigma and mental health
- Mental status findings (particularly speech and thought process)
- The role of rehabilitation

Final Analysis
Though this movie may not have made that many viewer's lists for highly recommended movies, it contains many educational gems, including:
- Pathological intoxication — valid entity or defense lawyer fabrication?
- The psychiatrist in court
- Ethical issues — can a psychiatrist begin a personal relationship with a patient's sister?
- Practice style — forensics blended with psychoanalysis?
- Dream theory and parapraxes (violets and violence)
- Malingering

Bandits
This movie nicely portrays the versatility that Billy Bob Thornton has as an actor, which varies over an incredible range of character types. In this film, he gives very accurate portrayals of two somatoform disorders: conversion disorder and hypochondriasis, as well as the sleeping disorder narcolepsy. The justifications he gives for his various ailments seems compelling, although it is done in a humorous fashion.

Reel to Real: Psychiatric Conditions in Cinema

Unstrung Heroes
This is a delightfully offbeat movie that contains a rich variety of portrayals. The main character is Steven Lidz (played by Nathan Watt). His father Sid (John Turturro) has obsessive-compulsive personality traits. Uncle Danny Lidz (Michael Richards) has paranoid personality disorder and literally explodes onto the scene at several points during the movie. Uncle Arthur Lidz has the residual subtype of schizophrenia and prominent negative symptoms. Steven's mother Selma (Andie MacDowell) develops cancer, so the family's adaptation to this illness is also an added educational element to this film.

Awakenings
This movie is based on a book by the same name written by the eminent neurologist Dr. Oliver Sacks. It features Robin Williams as Dr. Malcolm Sayer, and is a medically accurate portrayal of the aftermath of the encephalitis lethargica epidemic that occurred between 1917 and 1928. There are scenes that are terrific portrayals of catatonia and parkinsonian signs and symptoms, as well as other neurological conditions. In addition, many scenes have interesting and accurate portrayals of psychiatric symptoms.

He Love Me… He Loves Me Not
Shown from two distinctly different narratives, this French film is a masterful portrayal of erotomania. At first we see things from the "unreliable narrator" point of view, which comprises the main character Angélique's story of unrequited love. She is ostensibly having an affair with Dr. Loïc Le Garrec (Samuel Le Bihan). She is so charming and full of life that she wins the viewer over and one cannot help but wish the best for her in this ill-advised affair. Alas, it is not to be and the crestfallen Angélique attempts to take her life by asphyxiation. At this point, the film rewinds and shows things from an objective view, not just Loïc's perspective. The affair never existed. We were shown events completely out of context. Angélique did receive a flower from Loïc, but it was when he brought an arrangement home for his wife Rachel (Isabelle Carré) and he gave her one on a whim. Angélique was house sitting for Loïc and Rachel's neighbor, so he didn't go out of his way to meet her. This small act of kindness blossomed into a full-scale delusion on Angélique's part and consumes her life. She goes on to utterly devote herself to the prospect of life with Loïc, ignoring the opportunity to have a relationship with David (Clément Sibony). The ending to the film is a chilling reminder of the recalcitrant nature of erotomania.

All-Star Movie Recommendations

Zelig

This 1983 picture was years ahead of its time in terms of the technical aspects of reproducing the authentic newsreel look, and insinuating the main character Leonard Zelig (Woody Allen) in photos and historical film clips. Zelig is a human chameleon — a person so bereft of character that he not only assumes the attitudes of those he is around, he morphs physically to look like them as well. Zelig is seen with groups of people with various body shapes, skin colors, degrees of affluence, and political views and fits in seamlessly with them. Zelig was doing well left to his own devices, but once he became a medical and psychiatric curiosity, the attention and fame caused a variety of upsetting (but also hilarious) events to occur. This tendency to want to fit in so entirely with one's environment is an extreme form of an avoidant personality disorder. The film is also a great opportunity to discuss some of the historical elements of psychiatry, the roles and stereotypes of female psychiatrists, and the depiction of psychotherapy in film.

In a unusual case of life imitating art imitating life, there is actually a "Zelig-like syndrome" described in a patient who had anxoic damage to his frontal and temporal lobes (http://bps-research-digest.blogspot.com/2007/03/brain-damage-turns-man-into-human.html).

The Corporation

This movie is based on Joel Bakan's (2004) book by the same name. From nefarious beginnings, corporations have become today's dominant institution. By the end of the nineteenth century, through a bizarre set of legal alchemy, courts had fully transformed the corporation into a "person," with its own identity separate from the flesh-and-blood people who were its owners and managers, and empowered it like a real person to conduct business in its own name, acquire assets, employ workers, pay taxes, and go to court to assert its rights and defend its actions. After explaining how corporations became legal "persons," Bakan seeks to describe the corporation's character. He points out that the purpose of a corporation is to accumulate wealth for its shareholders — and nothing else. In outlining the pivotal law case of two automobile manufacturers, Bakan illustrates that social responsibility, while clearly beneficial, has been in fact deemed illegal because it is not in the best interests of the corporation. The movie then more fully describes the corporate character. The website for this project is http://www.thecorporation.com.

References

Alexander M, Pavlov A, Lenahan P
Cinemeducation: A Comprehensive Guide to Using Film in Medical Education
Radcliffe Publishing, Oxon, UK, 2005

American Psychiatric Association
Diagnostic and Statistical Manual of Mental Disorders, 4th Edition, Text Revision
American Psychiatric Association, Arlington VA, 2000

Bhagar HA
Should Cinema Be Used for Medical Student Education in Psychiatry?
Med Educ. 39(9): p. 972-3, 2005

Bhugra D
Mad Tales From Bollywood: The Impact of Social, Political, and Economic Climate on the Portrayal of Mental Illness in Hindi Films.
Acta Psychiatr Scand. 112(4): p. 250-6, 2005

Butler JR, Hyler SE
Hollywood Portrayals of Child and Adolescent Mental Health Treatment: Implications for Clinical Practice.
Child Adolesc Psychiatr Clin N Am 14(3): p. 509-22, 2005

Gabbard GO, Gabbard K
Psychiatry and the Cinema, 2nd Edition
American Psychiatric Publishing, Inc., Arlington VA, 1999

Gharaibeh NM
The Psychiatrist's Image in Commercially Available American Movies.
Acta Psychiatr Scand. 111(4): p. 316-9, 2005

Hesley JW, Hesley JG
Rent Two Films and Let's Talk in the Morning: Using Popular Movies in Psychotherapy, 2nd Edition
John Wiley & Sons, New York, 2001

References

Hyler SE
DSM-III at the Cinema: Madness in the Movies.
Compr Psychiatry 29(2): p. 195-206, 1988

Hyler SE, Gabbard GO, Schneider I
Homicidal Maniacs and Narcissistic Parasites: Stigmatization of Mentally Ill Persons in the Movies.
Hosp Community Psychiatry 42(10): p. 1044-8, 1991

Hyler SE, Schanzer B
Using Commercially Available Films to Teach About Borderline Personality Disorder.
Bull Menninger Clin. 61(4): p. 458-68, 1997

Robinson DJ
Reel Psychiatry: Movie Portrayals of Psychiatric Conditions
Rapid Psychler Press, Port Huron MI, 2003

Robinson DJ
Reel Psychiatry
International Journal of Psychiatry 21(3): p. 1-16, 2009

Schneider I
The Theory and Practice of Movie Psychiatry.
Am J Psychiatry 144(8): p. 996-1002, 1987

Solomon G
The Motion Picture Prescription: Watch This Movie and Call Me in the Morning: 200 Movies to Help You Heal Life's Problems
Aslan Publishers, Fairfield CT, 1995

Walter G, McDonald A, Rey JM, Rosen A.
Medical Student Knowledge and Attitudes Regarding ECT Prior To and After Viewing ECT Scenes From Movies.
J ECT 18(1): p. 43 - 46, 2002

Wedding D, Boyd MA, Niemiec RM
Movies And Mental Illness: Using Films To Understand Psychopathology, 2nd Edition
Hogrefer and Huber Publishers, Cambridge MA, 2005

Reel to Real: Psychiatric Conditions in Cinema

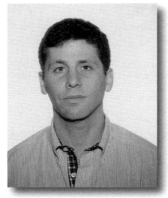

The Author
Dave Robinson is a psychiatrist practicing in London, Ontario, Canada. His particular interests are inpatient adult psychiatry, undergraduate and postgraduate education. He is a graduate of the University of Toronto Medical School and is a faculty member in the Department of Psychiatry at the University of Western Ontario.

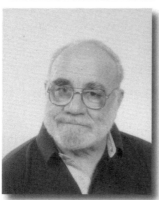

The Artist
Brian Chapman is a resident of Manitoulin Island, Ontario, Canada. He was born in Sussex, England and moved to Canada in 1957. Brian was formerly a Creative Director at MediaCom. He continues to freelance and is versatile in a wide range of media. Brian is married to Brenda, a fellow artist.

Rapid Psychler® Press

Rapid Psychler Press was founded in 1994 with the aim of producing textbooks and resource materials that further the use of humor in mental health education. In addition to textbooks, Rapid Psychler Press specializes in producing images for presentations.